Community Health Education

Community Health Education

Rameshwari Pandya

Rawat Publications

Jaipur • New Delhi • Bangalore • Hyderabad • Guwahati

ISBN 81-316-0343-1

Published by
Prem Rawat for **Rawat Publications**
Satyam Apts, Sector 3, Jawahar Nagar, Jaipur 302 004 (India)
Phone: 0141 265 1748 / 7006 Fax: 0141 265 1748
E-mail: info@rawatbooks.com
Website: www.rawatbooks.com

New Delhi Office
4858/24, Ansari Road, Daryaganj, New Delhi 110 002
Phone: 011 2326 3290

Also at *Bangalore, Hyderabad* and *Guwahati*

Typeset by Rawat Computers, Jaipur
Printed at Chaman Enterprises, New Delhi

Contents

Preface

Community Health Education is a very interesting and informative book. The author has put in all the shades and colours of health education into it. As a result, this book describes, explains, evaluates and even theorizes, wherever necessary, on the important issues of health and recreation as they apply to one and all. New and innovative teaching methods that have been used over the years for action projects and community outreach programmes in order to bring about social change are discussed in detail.

An amalgam of health and education, health education reflects the attributes of both and is committed to enhancing democratic learning processes, human dignity and community value systems. Health education can be defined as the area in which social and health sciences are applied to facilitate the development of healthy lifestyles and behaviour among people. It is important that the people in a community be organized to solve health problems through their own efforts in areas where no organized institutions are in action. This book profiles different projects such as the Health Club initiative conducted by Sarika Patel, the Tobacco Control project started by Janki Kothari and the Lifelong Education Programme of the Department of Extension and Communication, Faculty of Family and Community Sciences, MS University of Baroda, in Vadodara, Gujarat, and the Department's efforts to promote non-formal education among school dropouts, girls, women and elderly people in old age homes. Based on her experience in community outreach programmes, the author argues that the process of organization is an integral constituent in the process of lifelong learning.

The major objectives of the different projects that have been initiated thus far have been to impart education and conduct health and recreational activities. A combination of teaching and planned strategies, including charts, posters, flash cards, mobiles, *bhavai*, role play, street plays, puppets and focus group discussions were used to spread good healthy habits and impart both health education and recreation to people of the deprived sections of society because health and recreation play a vital role in the efforts to improve the lives of people living under adverse conditions. They play an important role in family, child and youth welfare, rural development and service to the elderly, the ailing and other individuals in need of special attention as they are the most vulnerable groups. They are weak and the most marginalized and often excluded from the purview of education programmes because their other needs take precedence over these. This book elaborates on some of the innovative methods that have been used to engage such people in a meaningful learning process that spans more than a decade. This book examines the potential of culturally and historically rooted action oriented educational methods and materials to address the problems of the deprived sections of people, women, children with special needs, and elderly people.

This book is based upon the author's belief that education has a larger canvas than literacy. Action itself can and should be used as a medium of education. The contents of such programmes should be related to social issues to make them meaningful and relevant to the lives of the learners. This book shows how these content areas can be addressed through action programmes. It will be useful to development workers, people working in government organizations and non-governmental organizations, graduate and postgraduate students of home science and women's polytechnics in universities and institutes of higher education. It will also serve the needs of activists, academicians, practitioners, policymakers and planners engaged in development management, who will definitely find this book stimulating and useful.

1 Adult and Non-Formal Education

What is a Community?

The term, 'community', concerns things held in common. They may be tangible, like the wealth of a family or the common pasture lands held by a tribe. Or, they may be intangible, as in common ideas, beliefs and values, common customs and norms, or the joint action of a group as a whole. Furthermore, when we speak of a community, ordinarily, we mean a set of people who do not constitute just one community in the larger society, as, for example, the adolescent community, the American African community and the academic community. The geographical clustering that constitutes a village, town or city ordinarily sets in motion certain processes that tend to make a community. One of the elements of commonness composing a community is similarity of activities. In any community where people are engaged in similar activities and are subject to the same or similar events, the very similarity generates topics for conversation, leads people to enjoy one another's company and creates bonds of mutual understanding.

What is Health?

Health is not mainly an issue of doctors, social services and hospitals. Health is a difficult term to define. All communities have their own concept of health. For some, it is "absence of disease". In some cultures, health and harmony are defined as "being at peace with the self, community, God and cosmos". According to Webster's Dictionary, health is "the condition of being sound in body, mind or spirit, especially freedom from physical diseases or pain". The World Health Organization (WHO) has attempted to construct a positive definition of health, describing it as "a state of complete physical, mental and social well-being and not merely the absence of disease or infirmity". Such a categorization of health is akin to a spectrum, with positive health at one end and a diseased state at the other end. This conceptualization permits one to talk of health as a dynamic state capable of moving up or down the ladder, rather than a static state in equilibrium. This is appropriate because health status cannot remain constant for an individual, family, community or country over a period of time.

Physical well-being can be easily understood by all of us. Physical health relates to the anatomical, physical and biochemical functioning of the human body. Thus, the attributes of physical health denote normalcy of the body structure and organs and their proper functioning. One should remember that a 'normal state' in medicine is based on the law of averages. The physical structure of the Cave Man or Ape Man may be considered abnormal in contemporary times, while it would be considered perfectly normal in the age in which these men lived. Various ways of assessing physical health are available, as, for example, height, weight, muscle mass and tests of bodily functioning such as forced expiratory volume, but all of them define normalcy in statistical terms and in relation to the risk of developing a particular disease.

Social well-being is more difficult to define. In its simplest connotation, social health means that level of health which enables people to live in harmony with their surroundings. Man is, after all, a social animal. He both learns from and contributes to society. Health is both a product and a determinant of social values. Cultural and ethnic background, traditions and mores, economic and literacy levels, needs and perceptions are all important in the consideration of social health. Social health can be measured, albeit indirectly, by attitude scales, socio-economic status, levels of literacy and employment status, among other indicators.

Mental well-being is perhaps the most abstract component to describe. Recent developments in psychiatry and psychology have helped in defining features of mental health in a better fashion. A positive, healthy mental state indicates that the individual enjoys his routine, there are no undue conflicts, bouts of depression or elevation of mood, and he has harmonious relations within the family and community.

Spiritual health may be considered a component of mental health. In societies such as India, religion has played an important role in shaping the cultural ethos. Many people believe strongly in the supernatural. In such situations, positive mental health embraces spiritual health. Spiritual health may help to resolve both internal and external conflicts.

Community Health

People can be healthy only when their surroundings are clean and pleasant, when the place where they live is clean and unpolluted. To be free from disease and to live a healthy life, they have to make their environment sound. In India, we find that many people suffer from disease due to poor and unhygienic living conditions, including lack of clean surroundings, all of which lead to poor health. Slums are one such place – the people living in slums are not very aware of the importance of cleanliness because they are less educated and have little knowledge about health. They live their lives blindly, accepting disease as part of their lives. They do not visit health centres, but try home remedies, which are not very effective. They take health issues lightly. They also do not have the money to treat their diseases and they suffer all through their lives, often dying prematurely.

The government offers many programmes to improve the health of slum dwellers, who are now being provided free health check-ups and free or subsidized medicines. They are being made aware of the importance of a clean environment and how it affects their health. Due to such programmes, we now see changes in the lifestyles of slum dwellers and that their health status and mortality rates have improved. We also find many non-governmental organizations (NGOs) working for the betterment of the health of slum dwellers and they have tried their best to make such communities realize that health is wealth.

Home scientists play an important and necessary role in the field of extension education. Their work is not limited to rural areas, it extends to urban areas as well; however, emphasis is placed on the development of the rural sector. Extension workers do multipurpose work. Home scientists are bound to touch upon all aspects of human life. They have comprehensive understanding of people and their problems. They should develop close contact with the people with whom they work and participate in their joys and sorrows. They should start their work with locally felt needs and win the enthusiastic cooperation of the people. Home scientists should help people choose a lifestyle that helps them to adjust to the society around them. They should respect the people's customs, traditions and ways of life, and create in them a willing spirit for real achievement. They must be a friend to the people and help them in all situations, even awkward ones.

As we know, India faces challenges on several fronts, prominent among them are poor health, poverty and illiteracy. Adult education provides the solution to most of these problems. Adult education is thus an imperative and overpowering need: All men and women must be helped to acquire the skills and knowledge that will enable them to fit properly into the fast-moving society around them. An illiterate person will face innumerable hurdles in this scientific and rapidly changing world of cut-throat competition. Literacy is not only a means of liberation, but also an instrument of social change. It is a tool for acquiring and sharing information on national development. Literacy increases people's capacity to cope with the demands of living and working. Adult education is a tool to influence human thinking in the right direction. In fact, the development of society depends primarily on the quality and effectiveness of its people. The importance of adult education in human resource development is being seriously recognized as an imperative for both economic development and for strengthening the base of democracy. The significance of universal literacy as an instrument for galvanizing and mobilizing people and arousing community consciousness and community participation for bringing about social change is also being acknowledged universally.

The Changing Concept of Adult Education

According to UNESCO, the term, 'adult education', denotes the entire organized education process – whatever the content level and method, whether or not it prolongs or replaces initial education in schools and college, and whether or not it includes apprenticeship – whereby persons regarded as adults by the society to which they belong, develop their abilities, enrich their knowledge, improve their technical or professional qualifications, and bring about changes in their attitude or behaviour in the two-fold perspective of full personal development and participation in balanced and independent social, economic and cultural development. Adult education programmes, as envisaged in the national adult education programme, are meant primarily for women and learners belonging to the deprived sections of society. This does not meant that others willing to join adult education programmes should be excluded, but that more attention must be paid to these sections of the population for they constitute about 60–70 per cent of India's population, and do not have the benefit of any type of education, whether formal or informal.

The report of the Kothari Commission for Education (1964–66) has this to say about the main concept of extension education: "This is not another scheme. This is not another co-curricular activity. It is the third dimension of the university system." The aim of extension is firstly to extend knowledge and institutes and resources to the community and vice versa. Its secondary aim is to gain insights from contact between knowledge resources and sociocultural realities, with a view to reflecting these insights in the entire curricular system of higher education, including teaching research.

Extension education is a two-way process, which encompasses 'college' and 'community'. It is the application of classroom knowledge to the community for the latter's benefit. People move towards development through awareness and assertion. People's participation is becoming an important issue in today's world. The slogan of a people centred and people controlled paradigm of development has acquired new urgency in the contemporary context. Education is closely associated with purposeful and organized social intervention programmes in the broader spectrum of human resource development. India has one of the largest educational networks in the world; ironically, it also has one of the largest number of illiterates.

Working in the Field

The Department of Extension and Communication, Faculty of Family and Community Sciences, MS University of Baroda (the city is now known as Vadodara), has been carrying out extension activities among different communities in Vadodara district for the last 50 years. Details of the major activities conducted by the Department in the last five years are given here:

Projects Undertaken

1. Survey of area
2. Literacy class
3. Innovative teaching aids
4. Environment education
5. Women's empowerment
6. Population education
7. Human rights
8. Health education
9. Reproductive health
10. Communal harmony
11. Moral education
12. Legal literacy
13. Income generation
14. Recreational activities

Slum areas in which the Department has worked:

1. Salatwada
2. Pensionpura
3. Jalaramnagar
4. Ektanagar
5. Makarpura, GIDC
6. Indira Nagar
7. Chhani Jakat Naka
8. Ajwa
9. Mali Mahola
10. Parsuram Bhatta
11. Fatepura
12. Sanjay Nagar

Teaching Aids

Different teaching aids such as mobiles, charts, posters, flash cards, flip charts, puppets, specimens and samples were used for conducting adult education and non-formal classes in slum communities for the Department's urban extension work.

Teaching Methods

Several innovative teaching methods were drawn up and used for contacting the community people and during the adult education and non-formal education classes. The important ones among these were demonstrations, workshops, plays, role play, educational games, discussions, expert talks and film shows, followed by discussions.

Methodology

Urban extension work is conducted with three specific objectives and with three different target groups.

The fieldwork is conducted by the final year students of the Department under the supervision of the teacher in-charge.

In the months from July to December, fieldwork is conducted in non-formal education with children and school dropouts from deprived communities. In the months from January to May, the target group is adult women. Since the last five years, the Department has also started work in the old age homes of Vadodara.

Under the Lifelong Education Programme, the MSc students train BSc students on how to plan, conduct and evaluate the programme. This has a dual purpose: The programme is well supervised by the senior students and, as a result, the quality of the programme is better; secondly, the senior students get trained in supervisory work, which is also an objective of the course.

Thus, the complete programme schedule encompasses:

- Non-formal education for children.
- Adult education for women.
- Lifelong education for senior citizens.
- Skills training courses, such as henna designs, embroidery and fabric painting for girls and women. These received an enthusiastic response from the community.
- Demonstrations and workshops on topics such as the use of jute products, creating soak pits, using water filters, letter holders and letter boxes, disseminating low cost recipes, teaching hair styling, stone painting and creating photo frames, and the creative use of waste.

- Recreational activities such as plays, *bhavai*, mono-acting, puppet shows, *garba*, Antakshari, indoor games, *bhajan-keertans* and picnics.

The community work is being carried out in different thrust areas, but here, I am providing a detailed description of only the community health projects undertaken by the Department.

Figure 1.1 *Approaches Used in Adult Education*

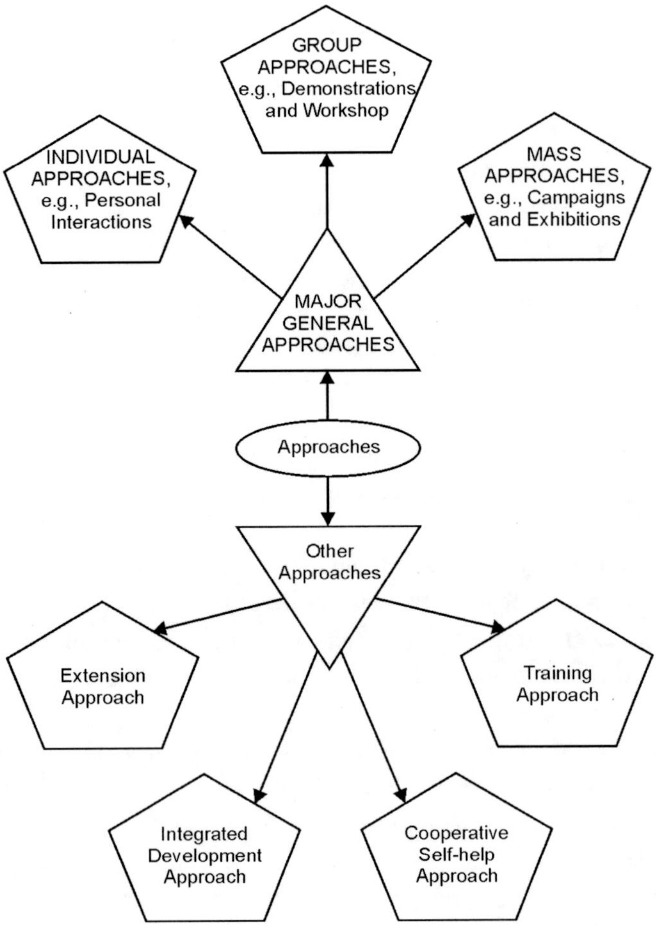

The Need for Community Health Education

1. To get the community involved in desirable health behaviour on the basis of the knowledge imparted.
2. To create a need in the community to work for the better health of its people.
3. To convince the community to contribute either in cash or in kind for the health and welfare of its people as and when needed.
4. To create public opinion through the community so that the government comes forward for the solution of health problems.
5. To get the community organized to solve health problems through its own efforts in areas where no organized institution, such as a municipality or corporation exists.

The Tasks of Health Educators

The task before health educators is to understand the community and its needs. They should possess adequate knowledge of the attitudes, customs, beliefs, prejudices, traditions and cultural patterns of the community so that they can fit modern scientific ideas of health into the existing structure. They should be able to assess the prestige and the power that a leader in the group enjoys and the leadership pattern in the community. As we all know, communication is a two way process and efficient communication ensures the success of any health education programme. Highly technical ideas need to be translated into a language which can be easily understood by the people for whom they are intended. Health educators, therefore, must be conversant with the methods and techniques of communication. The team of extension students and teachers at MS University of Baroda are well equipped to do this job.

The Role of Extension Workers

An old Chinese proverb says, "Outsiders can help, but insiders must do the job." This means that extension workers, usually community health workers, should be insiders who live in the community because only community members can understand local needs and traditions. Extension workers play a triple role in their community as health educators, health providers and agents of change.

- As educators, they teach the whole community how to improve health and prevent illness.
- As health providers, they warn against common illnesses early, before they become serious.
- As agents of change, they help community members change their knowledge, attitudes and practices so that they can lead healthier lives.

Extension workers carry out several tasks:

1. Making themselves available:
   They are willing to give appropriate care and advice to all community members, regardless of wealth, tribe, caste or religion, whenever needed.
2. Functioning as a teacher:
   They are continually passing on knowledge in a practical and helpful way whenever the opportunity arises, both to individuals and to groups.
3. Caring for children:
   (a) They help to promote good nutrition education. Extension workers measure the weight or mid upper arm circumference of children aged under five years once a month, filling in a growth chart or record card. They provide practical feeding advice to parents, emphasizing the value of breastfeeding and appropriate weaning. They help to arrange feeding programmes and set up kitchen gardens.
   (b) They demonstrate the use of oral rehydration therapy (ORT). This is a treatment for dehydration where oral rehydration salts (ORS) – either packed or prepared at home – are mixed with water and given to those suffering from diarrhoea. This special solution, which contains added sugar and salt, is life giving. So, such demonstrations help the community members know how and when to use ORT in the treatment of diarrhoea.

   (c) They promote the immunization of all children.
   (d) They distribute vitamin A and deworming medicines to children aged between one and five years in areas where these are health priorities.
4. Caring for mothers:
   (a) Extension workers promote prenatal care.
   (b) They motivate women to attend clinics for regular check-ups. They help in distributing iron and folic acid tablets to pregnant and lactating women and promote tetanus immunization.
   (c) They offer post-natal advice and care by organizing expert talks by doctors and nutritionists.
5. Promoting child spacing and family planning.
6. Caring for those with chronic infectious diseases, such as tuberculosis (TB), leprosy, HIV/AIDS and other locally significant diseases. This includes motivating patients for treatment and encouraging them to complete courses of medicine.
7. Caring for the blind, handicapped and disabled.
8. Giving illustrative talks on everyday illnesses and first aid.
9. Developing public health activities:
   Promoting hygienic waste disposal, vermicomposting, safe water, smokeless cooking hearths and other improvements to the home and environment, with the support of the health team or committee.
10. Working alongside their supervisors or other members of the health team. This may include taking part in surveys, immunization, caring for schoolchildren, teaching and supervision, health centre activities and community projects.
11. Forming community clubs:
   Setting up women's groups and promoting female literacy. They also develop health clubs, eco clubs, etc.
12. Encouraging parents to send their children to school
13. *Solving problems:* In the context of community health, the purpose of knowledge is to help find effective answers to practical problems. Larger projects, such as working in areas where clean water is a strongly felt need, help communities

develop new sources or make major improvements in storage or transport. Some examples:

(a) Running pipes from water sources to suitable sites in the community or into each house
(b) Drilling tube-wells or building new 'open' wells
(c) Installing hand pumps at existing wells

14. *Creating awareness:* A mother may know she should wash her hands before preparing food, but will not do so because no one has told her why it is necessary. Thus, she knows, but is not aware. Extension workers offer effective health teaching, supplemented by other teaching aids. For example, how to overcome drunkenness is shown well through puppet plays. The teaching is thus enjoyable, the audience feels involved and the message is clear in its dissemination. Flash cards are used to show the importance of family planning. Flip charts are used to show the different processes of water sterilization, by flannel graph, good health stories like those about immunization are prepared and practised using cut-outs.

    In role play, two people take on the roles of other people and act them out, as, for example, an extension worker talking to a TB patient, another talking to a pregnant woman, or a money lender talking to a poor villager. They use storytelling or singing, which are part of the local tradition.

    They also use live models to drive home their point. For example, when giving a talk on polio or malnutrition, they present before the audience a child who is actually disabled by polio or with obvious malnutrition (keeping in mind the sensitivities of the child and its parents). Such exercises help in making the health message more powerful.

    Posters in public places are used for emphasizing the necessity of maintaining a clean environment and planting trees. Plays are also used for creating awareness.

15. *Evaluating regularly:* This helps both extension workers and community members to focus their aims and direct their activities. Evaluation is necessary at regular intervals, especially when it is a part of an educational programme.

Impact

Impact is an expression of the overall effect of a programme, service or institution on the health status and socio-economic development of the targeted community. For example, as a result of the malaria control programme in India, not only has malaria incidence been reduced, but all aspects of life within the targeted communities – agricultural, industrial and social – have shown an improvement. If the target of 100 per cent immunization has been reached, it must also lead to reduction in the incidence of vaccine prevented diseases.

Impact on Students

Students who had enrolled for extension activities right from the beginning have experienced a change in their personalities. The feedback received from the Department's student volunteers encourages us to continue the task of community work. The work placement project has helped the students gain work experience and confidence to face a competitive world. The students reported that working in the communities was a new and pleasant experience. Some of the students reported that working with elderly people in old age homes gave them an insight into their problems and a new perspective on the lives of elderly people.

Impact on the Community

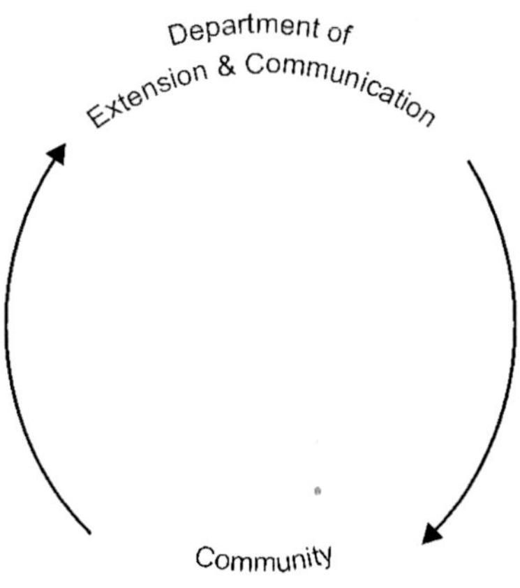

Different areas in and around Vadodara were adopted by the Department right from its inception. The people in these communities belong to different religions, castes and sex. They cooperated with us whole heartedly and, so, we could carry on all the activities we wanted, like the literacy project and surveys of women's status, population education and health

Figure 1.2 *Supervision in Adult Education*

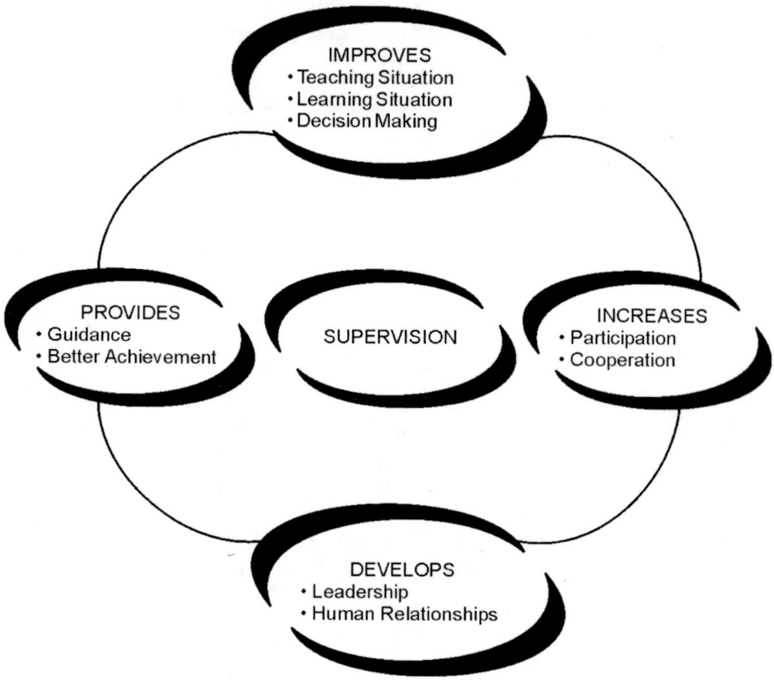

education. Thus, the Department, with the help of a dedicated team of teachers and students, has been successful in spreading knowledge. Education sharpens the eye of knowledge, develops awareness and makes the mind logical. Without proper education, the scope and extent of the processes of socio-economic change cannot be understood by common people and they are unable to participate in the process of development. Thus, we are contributing to the process of development.

Figure 1.3 *Guidance, Supervision and Evaluation of Students*

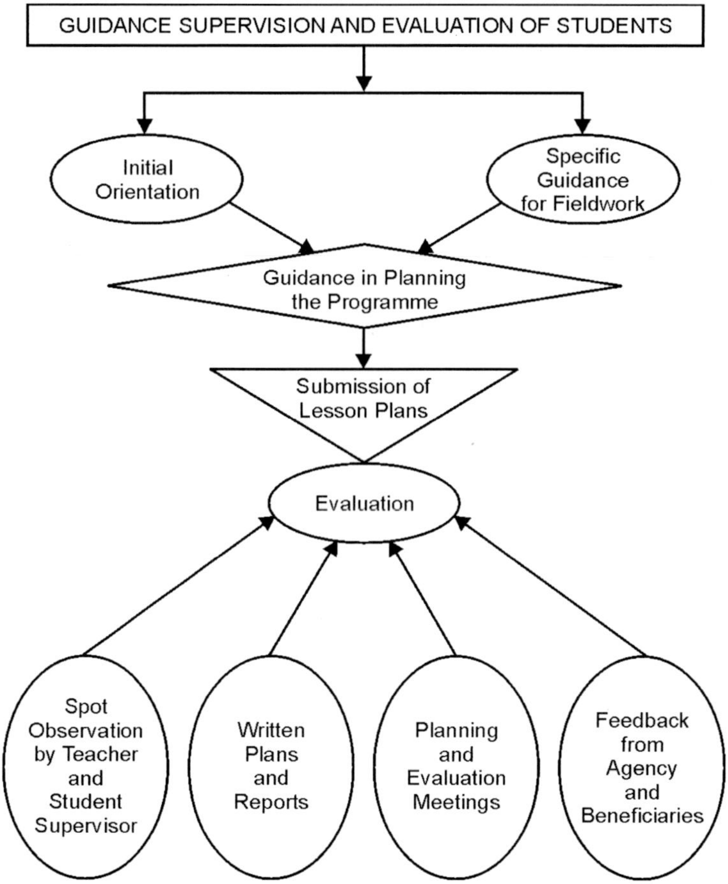

Bibliography

Ahuja, Ram. 1997. *Social Problems in India*. Rawat Publications, Jaipur.

Bhat, H.K. and Cheria, A. 1999. *Life Goes On: Sustainability of Community Development Programme and Withdrawal of Support*. Centre for Innovation, London.

Bhatia, S.C. 1980. *Some Critical Considerations in Adult Education*. Concept Publishers, New Delhi.

Desai, Vasant. 1988. *Rural Development*. Himalaya Publishers, New Delhi.

Dhama, O.P. 1985. *Education and Communication for Development*. Oxford University Press, New Delhi.

Dube, S.C. 2006. *India's Changing Villages*. Applied Publishers, New Delhi.

Gulati, R. and Gulati, K. 1999. *Strengthening Voluntary Action in India: Health and Family Planning Environment*. Konark Publications, New Delhi.

Human Development Report. 2003. 'Wonder Years in South Asia', in *The Times of India*, New Delhi, 12 December.

National AIDS Control Organization. 2000. 'Specialists' Training and Reference Module'. NACO, New Delhi.

Rehabilitation Council of India. 2004. 'Report on Manpower Development'. New Delhi.

2 Community Health Education

Issues and Perspectives

Health is fundamental to national progress. In terms of resources for economic development, nothing can be considered of higher importance than the health of the people, for it is a measure of their energy and capacity as well as of the potential man hours for productive work in relation to the total number of persons maintained by the nation. For the efficiency of industry and of the nation, the health of the worker as an essential consideration has been stated by the Planning Commission of India.

Health is viewed differently by different people all over the world. Health education is the sum of experiences that favourably influence habits, attitudes and knowledge relating to individual, community and racial health. Health education has been an integral part of the functions of health personnel since time immemorial – to educate people about the factors that influence their health. In the 20th century, we have been engaged in finding new technologies and medicines to tackle health problems.

People's behaviour needs to be moulded if they are to be made to understand and practise proper ways of living that will enable the maintenance of their health and avoid illnesses. Suitable education, which disseminates information about proper health practices, is required to ensure such moulding of behaviour. The process of persuading people to accept measures that will improve their health and to avoid those that will have an adverse effect is called health education.

Health education is a process that is carefully planned and effectively conducted with appropriate consideration of the ultimate good and the best means for reaching people. Although unplanned experiences contribute to an individual's education about health, health education is concerned with supplementing incidental experiences with those that are carefully related for their own values in attaining specific goals. Health education attempts to close the gap between what is known about optimum health practices and what is actually practised.

In addition to absence of disease, the concept of health includes knowledge, attitudes and behaviour that make it possible for people to live fully and happily. Health education includes quality of health, in which people have facts to learn, conclusions to draw, actions to take, and evaluations to make. Health, as a way of living as well as status, has to be earned and learned following certain well established concepts, norms and practices that may be gained through effective health education. Health education involves all those procedures designed to determine people's health status, to secure their cooperation in health protection and maintenance, to inform them of the diseases and defects that may be present in them, to prevent disease and to correct remediable defects. Basically, health education consists of procedures for presenting before people factual and important information regarding health and acquainting them with the various health, hygiene, sanitation and medical services and facilities that are available to them.

Public health is what people, as a society, do collectively to assure conditions in which they can be healthy. Health is a positive state of well-being in which harmonious development of the mental and physical capacities of people leads to the enjoyment of a rich and full life.

Health has found an important place in the constitutions of all countries and United Nations (UN) agencies. Of the 30 articles in the Universal Declaration of Human Rights, Article 25 is particularly concerned with the right to health. Everyone has a right to a standard of living adequate for the health and well-being of himself and of his family, including food, clothing, housing, medical care and necessary services, and the right to security in the event of unemployment, sickness, disability, widowhood, old age or other lack of livelihood, in circumstances beyond his control. Motherhood and childhood are entitled to special care and assistance. The preamble of the World Health Organization (WHO) constitution also states that enjoying the highest standards of health is a fundamental right of every human being and that governments are responsible for the health of their people.

What is Health Education?

The WHO Expert Committee on Health Education of the Public (1954) has defined health education in general is concerned with changes in the knowledge, feelings and behaviour of people. In its most usual form, it concentrates on developing such health practices as are believed to "bring about the best state of possible well-being".

The Need for Health Education

The working of the mind and the body are closely dependent on each other and neither can work efficiently if one or the other is not healthy. We know that prolonged lack of sleep or worry or mental troubles in young children can prevent their bodies from growing and developing in a normal way. Similarly, prolonged illnesses affecting the body, such as malaria or tuberculosis or weakness caused by malnutrition, will prevent the mind from being alert. If the mind is not alert, children cannot be expected to do well at their lessons. Repeated absences from school because of sickness further interfere with education. A principal cause of physical ill health is ignorance or neglect of health laws. The ability of people to produce enough food and secure the means of improving their living conditions depends largely on their state of health. A good system of education, therefore, should provide fully for the study of the laws of health and the teaching of healthy ways of living. The best time for this is during childhood, before thoughts and habits become fixed.

It is realized that ignorant parents and poor home surroundings may interfere to some extent with the health training given in schools. But it should be remembered that the school can benefit the community, not only by way of example of hygienic school buildings and teachers' homes and the observance of hygienic practices within the school, but through the active cooperation of teachers and pupils in the health and social activities of the community that the school serves.

Health education helps people to develop the knowledge and skills to undertake activities that will enable them to help themselves in achieving optimal health. People must understand the nature and purpose of the health services and facilities provided to them so that they can make the best use of these. Health education improves the health status of individuals, families, communities, states and the nation.

Health education enhances the quality of life for all people. By focusing on prevention, health education reduces the costs – both financial and human – that individuals, employers, families, insurance companies, medical facilities, communities, the state and the nation would spend on medical treatment. A close look at current trends shows that health education within the school and in the broader community outside the school are far more similar. Today, health educators have very similar goals and procedures, which are altered only by the type of setting in which the education is being conducted. In this respect, the relationships between school health education and community health education are many. In addition to these many similarities, there are several other ways in which school health education programmes relate to community health.

School health educators should be aware of the many people working in community health agencies who can be used for planning, dealing with special problems, and as general and specific resource personnel.

Since the school is a part of the community, school health educators should cooperate with community efforts in areas such as educational programmes and prevention of specific health problems.

School health educators need to let community agencies know what is going on in their school educational programmes. Both school and community health workers can best accomplish their goals by cooperating with each other. People working in community health agencies may have expertise in specific subject matter areas that are a part of the health curriculum. They may be able to help plan that part of the curriculum or even come to the school to make a presentation to the students. From time to time, special school problems might arise related to the concerns of some community agencies. With the wide range of voluntary health agencies concerned specifically with heart disease, cancer, birth defects, the respiratory system, family planning and nutrition, it should be possible to find experts in many areas of the curriculum. Usually, personnel in voluntary agencies also have the most recent information about their particular area. These resources are in addition to those that might be found in a state or local health department.

Related to, but still somewhat different from the preceding ideas is the fact that the school's presence as part of the community gives it a responsibility to cooperate with community health efforts. In a given community, there may be emphasis upon immunization, environmental problems or promotion of individual awareness of specific health concerns. School health educators may be able to enhance the efforts of community personnel by including appropriate material in the health curriculum, even though it may necessitate covering topics in an order that is different from the master plan. The compensation for this adjustment will be that the community emphasis will help make the learning experience better for the students.

School health educators need to remember that the school educational programme does not operate effectively in a vacuum. It is appropriate and necessary to continually let community agencies know what is happening in the school programme. This is not only good public relations, but could easily lead to a better educational programme. Community personnel might be aware of subject matter or have useful ideas, which remain inappropriate if school health educators do not keep them informed. This is a good example of a two way street, since community personnel may see a need to alter their programmes based on what is going on in the school. Cooperation will help both community segments to reach their similar goals in a better and more meaningful manner.

The Meaning of Community Health Education

One of the greatest difficulties confronting teachers, students or the public is the lack of a precise definition of the words and terms used to convey the ideas of disease and health. These difficulties seem to multiply with the increase in the literature dealing with prevention medicine, public health and health education. Because the phrase, 'community health education', contains words that are relative in character, it behoves health educators to be definite in the way the words are used in day-to-day discussions.

The most recent definition suggested by the Committee on Hygiene and Public Health, Delhi (2002): "Public health is the art and science of maintaining, protecting and improving the health of the people through organized community effort. It includes the arrangements whereby the community provides medical services for special groups of persons and is concerned with prevention or control of disease, with persons requiring hospitalization to protect the community."

An example of the difficulty in precise definition is the word, 'community'. A community may be defined as a form of social organization that meets certain human needs. Upon examination of this definition, it is revealed immediately that 'human needs' may be geographic in terms of land area, political in the system of laws governing the group, social in the opportunities afforded for social intercourse, economic in the dominant process for earning a livelihood, and psychological in the degree to which a group may be like-minded. Commonly used, these basic connotations are complicated further when we add the adjectives 'urban', 'suburban', 'rural', 'agricultural', 'industrial' and 'educational'. The problem becomes even more intricate when we use the phrase, 'community health education'. It becomes necessary to agree upon a definition of each of the component words – 'community', 'health' and 'education'. When we examine the word, 'health', we find ourselves in the same situation as in using the word, 'community'. Health comes from the Anglo-Saxon word, 'health', which means 'whole'. Wholeness is that quality of life in which the body is sound, the various organs function naturally and the whole organism responds adequately to its environment.

Basically, the struggle for social security, which, until about a hundred years ago, was an individual responsibility, is one directed by the community against the destructive powers of ignorance, disease and poverty. Other names for these destructive forces are illiteracy and poverty. The control of these destructive forces, which are age old in their pressures upon man, has yielded under the impact of individual and community education.

Aims and Objectives of Health Education

The main aim of health education is to help people achieve health by their own actions and efforts. Health education begins, therefore, with the interest of people in improving their conditions of living and aims at developing a sense of responsibility for bettering their own health as individuals and as members of a family and community.

To Make Health a Valued Community Asset

The value placed on health by people depends mainly on social and cultural factors such as the needs, problems, social organizations, standard of general education, and the economic resources of the people for individual, family and community betterment.

To Help Individuals to Become Competent

Health is not a commodity which can be bought by people for their improvement. They have to accept scientific knowledge, in particular that pertaining to health, and act accordingly. Therefore, the family and community should take responsibility for their own health.

To Promote the Development and Proper Use of Health Services

The usefulness of any health services provided by a health agency depends on the people's utilization of the services. It depends upon the confidence of the people in the health personnel and the attitudes which health workers have towards the people. By educating people, one can avoid the economic loss incurred by wrong or inadequate use of health services. Health education is an essential component of any programme to improve the health of a community and it plays a major role in promoting the following:

- Good health practices: For example, sanitation, clean drinking water, good hygiene, infant feeding and oral dehydration.
- The use of preventive services: For example, immunization, screening, antenatal and child health clinics.
- The correct use of medication and the pursuit of rehabilitation regimens: For example, in tuberculosis and leprosy, respectively.
- The recognition of early symptoms of disease and promoting referrals.
- Community support for primary health care and government control measures.

Principles of Health Education

The understanding of health education will be aided by a review of certain facts and principles that underline the development and administrative conduct of the programme.

An individual's health is determined by both heredity and mode of living. Because of the differences in their constitutions, two children with the same programme of living may not maintain the same levels of health.

Health education is by and large in the hands of elementary school teachers. Repetition plays a crucial role in the modification of habits and this should be recognized. Children form habits, not by learning facts, but by doing things repeatedly with satisfactory results.

Health education must be accepted and fostered by the administrative authorities as a part of the educational programme if it is to succeed. It is impossible for a teacher to develop a real health education programme without the support of the principal, the general supervisors, and the superintendents or inspectors of education, and physical education and health. It is certainly impossible for a teacher to develop a well organized programme without such support.

Effective health education demands the understanding, sympathy, cooperation and support of health specialists in the school system. Physicians, nurses, dentists, physical educators and nutritionists understand the value of their contribution and cooperation in health education programmes. Criticism, discussion and inaction will weaken even the best programme. The experience of medical examinations, physical inspections and dental corrections can be made more meaningful by schoolteachers. Children who know that health facts are measurable by their age and grade and are conditioned to practise good health habits will be desirous of taking the fullest advantage of the opportunities for learning more about their health status. These children will also be more cooperative in securing the necessary correction of any physical defects. Before acting upon medical advice from medical personnel, schoolchildren are stimulated by the force of social approval in the classroom to obtain corrections with a minimum of follow-up.

It is necessary for children to develop health practices before they are old enough to understand the scientific basis for the practices. Practice is needed before education starts. Health training begins at home, and it is supplemented at school. Health training should be organized from the very lowest grade. As children grow, knowledge upon which health practices are based should be presented progressively, according to their interest and capacity. Pupils begin school with the acceptance of a few fundamental health habits, the value of which they do not question. They finish their school education with an intelligent application of the fundamental principles of health to their own particular needs and activities.

Correct attitudes are important. The desirable attitude towards health regards it as a means of enriching life and not as an end in itself. Health contributes happiness, comfort, joy and maintenance of social relationships. It also contributes to the accomplishment of the fundamental aims of life. It is sought for what it helps us to be and to do so. Health is the means towards such fundamental objectives as characters, citizenship and service.

All children can succeed to some degree in improving health practices. The recognition of individual successes and the provision for every child to participate in health activities is a long stride towards making the programme enjoyable. In the development of any health habit, the teacher is, of course, concerned with the development of specific attitudes that will help children recognize the value of health and their desire to practise the strategies that lead towards it.

Functions of a Health Education Programme

Change in Knowledge

The most important need that a health education programme can serve is to provide appropriate knowledge about health and diseases to people. This knowledge should be provided in such a way that the recipients do not find it hard to accept. How can this knowledge be provided in an acceptable way? This is the first challenge faced by a health educator.

Change in Attitude

A change in attitude is possible only when the new knowledge that is offered is acceptable to the recipients. Its utility should also be well known to them. Normally, provision of appropriate knowledge should lead to the formation of positive attitudes, not only towards a person's own health, but also towards the health of other members of the community.

Change in Behaviour

Once positive attitudes are formed, these must reflect in the behaviour of the recipients. They should not only become mindful of their past behaviour, but should also avoid doing things which can in any way influence occurrence or spread of diseases.

Change in Habits

The change in the behaviour of the recipients must lead to habit formation. A habit can be formed only when the behaviour becomes repetitive. If proper habits are formed, not only the individuals concerned, but the whole community also will be benefited.

Change in Customs

Acquisition of positive attitudes leading to appropriate habit formation must sooner or later evolve into customs. Only when a substantial number of people in a given cultural setting start behaving in a customary manner can one say that the behaviour has become a part of their customs.

This process may be directed towards the following important programme elements:

- Personal hygiene
- Knowledge of modern medicine
- Nutrition
- Mental health
- Prevention of communicable diseases
- Care of children
- Environmental sanitation
- Human physiology
- Lifestyle diseases
- Education about alcohol and drugs
- HIV/AIDs and sexually transmitted diseases (STDs)

The organization of communitywide programmes of health education is, therefore, a complex matter requiring special knowledge and special skills. It cannot be left to the marginal attention of an already overworked medical officer or education officer. The people in charge of such programmes need to carry out periodic surveys of the health knowledge, habits and attitudes of the community; to plan and execute the educational work indicated by such surveys; to bring into this work all the many official and voluntary agencies which can contribute to it; to arrange, in cooperation with the professional groups concerned, special 'refresher' courses for doctors, nurses, teachers, caterers and so on; to organize an advice bureau and to maintain a liaison between that and the already existing specialist advisory centre; to prepare, assemble, display and distribute health education material of all kinds; and to do all this without treading on the many sensitive issues that usually surround such information.

As the importance of careful planning of community health education becomes increasingly appreciated, the need arises for the recognition of a new occupation – that of the 'health educator'. Already, national and local government agencies have made many such appointments and there have been several successful experiments. Successful health educators will require – apart from considerations of personality and general culture – basic training in the science of health, in the psychology and methods of education, the social sciences, and in public relations and administration.

Special training at present ranges from attendance at a single short conference to participation in comprehensive courses and summer schools, and its value is not to be minimized. Teachers who are sacrificing part of their well-earned vacations and social workers who are worried about what is happening in their area while they are away, cannot reasonably be expected to give the time and effort needed for a really fruitful study of the problems and potentialities of health education. It is, therefore, to be hoped that before very long, arrangements will be made to allow such persons leave of absence for periods of a month or more, so that they may pool their experiences and ideas. We are gradually filling the biggest gap in our corps of teachers, while health and social workers are increasingly coming within the framework of national and local governments, and it ought soon to be possible to second representatives to attend study courses.

Each professional group already has ample opportunity for intellectual inbreeding; it is the effect of cross-fertilization that is most lacking. One can imagine (and, unfortunately, we are as yet largely limited to imagination) how much matter of value would emerge from a month's cooperative study by a mixed group of parents, teachers, youth leaders, doctors, health visitors, administrators and social others, and how many pet notions each group would have to discard! There would be little need for 'expert' lecturers for what extra knowledge each group needed could probably be supplied by another and what greater understanding would emerge for all of them from their joint discussions. Unfortunately, most of us are so wedded to the traditional procedure of listening to lectures, and some of us so love having others to lecture to, that the idea of such a 'working party' bears a tinge of utopianism.

What this comes to, in effect, is a plea for the democratization of health education. Excellent work has been done in the past by socially minded doctors, health minded educationists and educationally minded social workers, but each group has tended to remain in its own special field. Yet, democracy involves not only doing one's own special job well, but also cooperating with other specialists as fellow citizens in communal tasks, and here, in health education, is a job for the whole community – a job which will not be well done until all natural health educators breakthrough the boundaries between their separate fields, place their specialist tools at each other's disposal, and till the great new common field together.

The Role of Home Scientists

Home scientists can play a significant role in the promotion of health education.

As teachers, home scientists can impart health education to both students and the community. Since teachers are respected by the youth and their parents, they wield considerable influence among the rural population in general. Since they are considered knowledgeable people, their advice carries credibility and conviction among the clients.

As researchers, home scientists can conduct various research studies and find out the needs of health education, the areas in which it needs to be imparted, and ways to impart it.

As extension workers, home scientists can promote health education in both urban and rural areas by organizing workshops, debates, seminars, expert talks, etc.

Conclusion

Health education aims at enabling people to gain "control over the determinates of health and health behaviour and the conditions that affect their health situation and the health status of others". Advances in human ecology have found that health is not only the result of the interaction of man with his biological environment, but also with his physical, chemical and social environments. Decisions and actions by various sectors of society do influence the health and living conditions of not only people belonging to that sector, but that of society as a whole. Health education has, therefore, to play a key role in influencing all health related sectors and in ensuring that their policies and actions are in congruence with national health objectives. It has also to play an advocacy role to see that such actions become possible.

Many developmental agencies that have contact with the people can also play an effective role in educating their clients in adopting sound health practices. Health educators, with limited resources at hand, have therefore to build partnerships with such developmental agencies so as to plan and implement coordination efforts towards empowering people with the knowledge and skills that will enable them to take responsibility for their own health and that of their community. Health education is, therefore, not only a means for action coordination, but is equally benefited by such action.

In conclusion, it can be seen that the goal of health for all can be achieved only by:

- Establishing full-fledged primary health care centres in all villages to look after all the health and medical needs of the people, taking each family as a unit.
- Reorganizing the present health and medical services in order to make it people oriented, need-based and rules oriented.
- The unmated control of all the health services will be exercises as central authority level, from where the needed administrative delegation of authority will be given downwards till the village level to supervise, manage, monitor and control all health and medical activities.
- Placing more emphasis on different health programmes and policies according to the target group.
- Integrating health services with international organizations.
- Engaging the active involvement of public and voluntary organizations.
- Monitoring, evaluating and auditing health activities at the national level.
- Working out broad based administrative policies and strategies.

- Giving more importance to research, professional ethics and standards, and working with dedication in line with the latest developments.

Bibliography

Bharadhwaj, R.K. 1974. *Urban Development in India*. National Publishing House, Delhi.

Bhattacharya, V.R. 1976. *Communication in a Global Village*. Chetna Publishers, New Delhi.

Bijlani, H.V. 1980. *Urban Problems*. IIDA, New Delhi.

Census of India. 1991. 'Ageing Population of India: Analysis of the 1991 Census Data'. Registrar General of India.

Kamat, Prasad. 1988. *Planning the Grassroots*. Sterling Publishers, New Delhi.

Park, J.K. 2000. *A Textbook of Preventive and Social Medicine*. Rawat Publications, Jaipur.

Pejaver, R.K. and Nair, M.K.C. 2001. *Adolescent Care 2000 and Beyond*. Prism Books Ltd., Bangalore.

3 Population Education

Need of the Hour

India is the second most populous country in the world, with more than 16 per cent of the world's population on 2.4 per cent of the land area. India's population has increased from 361.1 million in 1951 to 846.3 million in 1991, although the average annual exponential growth rate decreased for the first time after independence in 1947 to 2.14 during 1981–91. Despite some efforts to arrest its growth rate, the Indian population is increasing rapidly by about 17 million every year.

Against this background of population dynamics in India, population education and family life education for adolescents, young couples and adults assume special importance. The world population was more than six billion in 2000 with almost 90 per cent of the growth taking place in the developing countries. According to the 1981 Census of India, the country's population was 683.81 million, growing at an annual rate of 2.21 per cent. United Nations (UN) estimates show that the population of India in mid-1988 was 818.78 million; the estimates say this will increase to 1,455.57 million by 2025.

There are two main reasons inter alia for the hidden momentum of population growth in developing countries. These are (i) the sociocultural and religious values of the people, which influence their fertility behaviour, and (ii) the large young population of these countries. Population change is both a biological and a sociocultural phenomenon. The whole process of reproduction, leading to the birth of a child, is biological. But, the decisions behind the birth of a child and the size of a family are governed by sociocultural values, traditions and customs.

At the time of the World Population Conference in 1974, representatives from many countries argued that the best form of contraception was economic development. The conventional wisdom at the time assumed that once developing economies improved, a 'demographic transition' would be automatic. Many countries have since modified their assumptions. One reason for this turnaround in thinking was the intrusion of reality: No such automatic process took place. In addition, information campaigns launched by the United Nations Population Fund (UNFPA), non-governmental organizations (NGOs) and other development agencies demonstrated that developing and using population and development programmes can provide the key to lower fertility rates. In this task, the media played, and will continue to play, a paramount role. Although editors and writers have periodically rediscovered 'population issues' over the last 35 years, they are still regarded as a 'soft' topic. Nevertheless, the mass media are giving increasing space to the connections linking population issues to environmental and developmental concerns. One of the reasons for this is that the UNFPA's State of World Population report has received worldwide media attention. More than 1,000 publications around the world ran articles, features and editorials on the 1993 State of World Population report, and 400 radio and television stations broadcast special programmes based on material from the report and interviews with population experts. Journalists and editors are becoming more sensitized to the subject of population growth and its relationship with sustainable management of the earth's resources.

Specialized coverage of population issues has also improved. A number of popular forums now exist, through which population and family planning issues can be disseminated to a wider, non-specialized audience. They fund their own monthly magazines, with readership estimated at more than 1,00,000 and provide coverage of population and family planning issues to an international audience. In addition, population issues are aired through the annual World Population Day, sponsored by the UNFPA, which includes information and educational activities, including an international poster competition for schoolchildren.

India's enormous and rapidly increasing population is perceived as a great strain on its natural resources and ecological environment and a formidable obstacle in its economic development. India has made consistent efforts towards development and modernization through its Five-Year Plans, in which the periodic review and revision of its population policy to reduce the rate of population growth has become an integral part of socio-economic development. The Eighth Five-Year Plan focused primarily on social determinants such as female literacy, age at marriage, and creation of employment opportunities for women to help improve their status in society. These factors are considered as important as achieving a reduction in infantmortality, improving the health and nutrition of primary schoolchildren and providing a comprehensive package of maternal health care services. We need to study the development phasewise if we wish to gain a better understanding about it. So far, three phases of the family planning project have been completed.

First Phase (1987–93)

The focus of the activities during the first phase – from 1987 to 1993 was to integrate well-identified messages, namely, small family norm, responsible parenthood, right age at marriage, population growth and environment, taking beliefs and traditions into account in teaching and learning materials. Based upon these messages, motivational, instructional and follow-up materials were brought out in the training curricula of adult education functionaries.

Second Phase (1994–98)

The second phase of the project from January 1994 to May 1998 was directed towards the goals set forth in the National Literacy Mission. It also reflected the priorities set out by the nodal agency, the Ministry of Health and Family Welfare (MHFW). The districts identified by the MHFW as having high infant mortality rates, disproportionate sex ratios, high crude birth rate, and low mean age at marriage were given precedence during this phase. The other dimensions focused on were related to information, education and communication (IEC) activities in the emerging areas of national concern – areas such as gender bias, inter-spouse communication, sexually transmitted diseases (STDs), HIV/AIDS, etc.

Third Phase (1998–2001)

The third phase of the project ran from June 1998 to December 2001. In view of the high rate of participation of women in the literacy programme and also realizing the significance of women's role in ensuring better quality of life, issues related to women's empowerment, gender equality, reproductive health and rights, family life education, and sexual health education were given an added thrust.

Population Education and Its Relationship with Health

Earlier it was felt that sex information should be withheld from children and adolescents and given only to young adults as they prepared for marriage. This feeling grew out of a popular fear that giving information about sex to children would stimulate their curiosity and lead to precocious sexual experiences. In order to avoid being misunderstood, we must point out that the goal of these methods of population education was good. We need methods that will achieve the goals of the yesteryears and at the same time lay the foundation for a happy and wholesome family life in later years in our children. It has been realized that there is a close relationship between the population situation, available resources, environment and development. There is an urgent need to maintain a balance between these factors. Unless the goal of population stabilization is attained and consumption levels rationalized, the environment will continue to be adversely affected. It is generally agreed that human beings, and not human numbers, should be the centre of all population and development activities. Apart from food, shelter and clothing, two other traditionally identified basic needs are health and education. Other primary needs now identified are employment and assets, which provide a certain degree of economic security. Health includes issues such as nutrition, expectation of life at birth, maternal and child health care, especially care of the girl child, immunization and reproductive health.

Many biological, social and cultural factors influence women's status in societies. Early marriage, early and frequent child bearing, and food taboos during pregnancy are some of the associated health risks as established by various field studies. Improving women's reproductive health is essential for improving their general health and it is also the basis for women's empowerment and one of the foundations of social and economical development. Good reproductive health among women is essential for the early stabilization of the world's population.

The 1994 Cairo International Conference on Population and Development (ICPD) emphasized that improving reproductive health, including adoption of family planning practices, is essential to human welfare and development. The ability of parents to choose the number, time and spacing of their children is considered an essential component of reproductive health. At the same time, the high worldwide incidence of STDs and HIV/AIDS among people, particularly among women and young children, are posing threats to the entire health management system.

What is Population Education?

Several people have attempted to define the concept of population education. Some of these definitions are presented here:

In 1971, a Ford Foundation expert defined it thus: "Population education is the educational process by which the reason of attitudes towards small family size is brought about. Population education is merely an instruction in the dynamics of population without the emotionally charged areas of sex, birth control and family planning. Population education is a moulder of attitudes and creator of predispositions to plan families of a reduced size. It is consisted of family planning and birth control; its role is long range and its approaches are interdisciplinary, multilevel and continuing."

UNESCO (1974) regards population education, not as a programme of propaganda or indoctrination, but as an educational approach intended to bring about an understanding of population phenomena. This implies that in the classroom, population change is not seen automatically as a 'problem'. Students are allowed to decide for themselves, after studying and discussing the relevant data, whether the population situation in their community, nation or the world at large can be identified, whether its nature should be clarified, and encouraged to explore a variety of possible solutions. Teaching methods which promote enquiry, analysis and active student participation in the discussions are essential to this new form of education, the content of which must be relevant to the students' needs and must also prepare them for the unknown, namely, a world situation, which, within a few years, will be very different from that of today.

According to V.K.R.V. Rao, "population education is no more than a part of the whole subject of human resource development and it should be treated as such both in content and in exposition". It is also essential that in the treatment of each of these items, population should not be treated merely as a quantitative phenomenon that is most relevant both as a factor of growth and an end product of growth and numbers have to be treated in terms of the effect they have on quality, either by way of deterioration or of improvement.

In a national workshop-cum-seminar on population education, T.S. Mehta defined population education as "an educational programme, which provides for a study of the world, with the purpose of developing in the students, national and responsible attitudes and behaviours towards the situation".

Broadly, population education can be defined as an educational programme which provides for a study of the population situation in a family, community, nation and the world, with the purpose of developing in the students a rational and responsible attitude and behaviour towards that situation. The objective of population education is to enable students to understand that family size is controllable, that population limitation can facilitate the development of a higher quality of life in the nation, and that a small family size can contribute materially to the quality of living for the individual family. It should also enable students to appreciate the fact that for preserving the health and welfare of the members of the family, to ensure the economic stability of the family and to assure good prospects for the younger generation, the Indian families of today and tomorrow should be small and compact.

The term, 'population', for the purpose of education, can be defined as the people living in a specified geographical area, be it a village, taluka, district, country or the world. Education is the process that imparts, improves or changes the knowledge, information, understanding, attitudes, skills, abilities, practices and so on of the people for their effective performance in life as an individual and as a member of a family, society and nation.

Population education is an educational programme that helps learners to understand the interrelationship of population dynamics and other factors of quality of life and to make informed and rational decisions with regard to population related behaviour with the purpose of improving the quality of life of themselves, their families, communities, nations and the world.

In all the definitions, the common objectives or purposes of population education are to:

Understand the prevailing population situation, the dynamic forces that have shaped it and the effect it will have on the present and future welfare of the people, their families, their communities and the world.

Make conscious and informed decisions based on people's understanding and evaluation of situations in their interest and that of others.

An educational programme aims to develop in the learner, understanding of the interrelationship between population and quality of life.

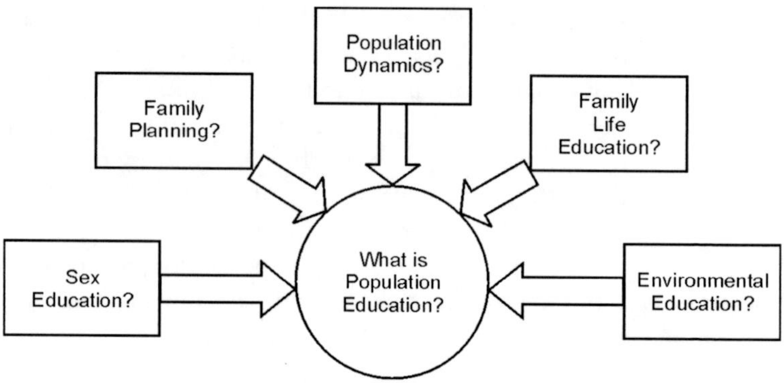

Objectives of Population Education

As in the case of the definition of population education, there has been considerable divergence in the objective content and scope of such education. Population education was instituted in response to the recommendations of the World Plan of Action, which stated that governments should consider making provisions in both formal and non-formal education programmes to inform their people of the consequences of both the existing and alternate fertility behaviour on the well-being of the family, on the educational and psychological development of children, and on the general welfare of society so as to promote an informed and responsible attitude towards marriage and reproduction.

Nevertheless, in view of the different socio-cultural backgrounds and population policies of the various countries, the specific objectives of population education are different in different countries.

The major objectives of population education are:

- To develop an understanding of demographic concepts and processes.
- To develop among the younger generation an understanding of the most important phenomenon of the modern world.
- To develop an understanding of the influence of population trends on the various aspects – cultural, political and economic – of human life.
- To develop an understanding of the close interaction of population growth and the developmental process with particular reference to development programmes for raising people's standard of living.
- To develop an understanding of the evil effects of overpopulation on the environment and the concomitant dangers for the population.
- To develop an understanding of the biological factors and phenomenon of reproduction, which are responsible for the continuation of the species.

- To develop an attitude of responsibility and mutual help and cooperation in all aspects of personal and family living.
- To develop an awareness of the population policies and programmes of the country.
- To provide students with basic demographic material and some understanding of it.
- To develop an appreciation of (i) the small family norm as proper and desirable, (ii) the relationship between population size and quality of life, and (iii) the fact that family size is a matter of deliberate choice and human regulation, rather than of accident or forces beyond human control.

There should also be awareness of the health risks involved in child bearing for both the mother and the child. Appreciation of the small family as a setting in which high quality of life for each person is more likely to be attained is another objective. In view of the different sociocultural backgrounds and population policies of the various countries in the world, the specific objectives of population education programmes are different for different grade levels and different target groups.

Goals of Population Education

The role of education is to endow learners with the kinds of tools that will help them understand the various aspects of any given phenomenon. This is precisely the goal that population education sets for itself, it proposes to help learners to define and understand the nature and causes of phenomena and their interrelationships with the realities of economic, social and cultural development.

Involving students in this learning process would not only enable them to understand population related issues, but also put them in a position where they would be able to make 'better informed decisions on population related matters, which would be personally meaningful and socially relevant'. This means that instead of the student being presented with a readymade course of action, his decisions would be developed during the process of learning.

What to Teach in Population Education?

"Population education, being of recent origin, has no clearly marked content boundaries; it is interdisciplinary in nature and related to various subjects. The problem of overcrowded curricula makes it difficult to establish population education as an independent subject in schools. The countries have, therefore, used an integration approach to include population education concepts in different subject areas. The National Seminar on Population Education held in Mumbai in August 1996 recommended the integration approach and the arguments presented in its favour were: The curriculum is already overcrowded and the demands of traditional subjects are increasing because of the explosion of knowledge. Children will probably learn more if they are confronted with relevant population material. Although the integration approach is being used by all the Asian countries that are running population education programmes, its purposefulness is being debated because of which some countries have started thinking of introducing it as a separate subject in schools.

Interrelationship among Factors Affecting Quality of Life

Population education is an innovation that spans distance and time and it encompasses a survey of the past, both distant and recent, the immediate present, and the near as well as distant future. In this sense, it spans time in a unique manner. Another innovative feature of population education is its relevance to problems and issues and the consequent life decisions that are important for every individual. It, therefore, challenges students to develop creative thinking and action in relation to these issues by providing an insight into the complexities of marriage, family size, number of children, spacing of children, health of the mother, pregnancy, risks, and so on. The thrust areas for material and training are:

- Small family norms.
- Responsible parenthood.
- Right age at marriage.
- Population growth and environment.
- Population and development.
- Beliefs and traditions.

- Gender bias.
- Inter-spouse communication.
- Women's empowerment.
- Reproductive health and reproductive rights.
- Fostering human dignity.
- Adolescent reproductive health and reproductive rights.
- Family life education.
- Preventive and curative education for STDs and HIV/AIDS.
- Sex education.
- Economic development and population.
- Social development and population.
- Health, nutrition and population.
- Biological factors, such as family life and population.

These can be dealt with in detail in the syllabus of various subjects, such as social studies, environmental studies, general science, mathematics and languages, into which it can be integrated at the elementary and secondary school levels.

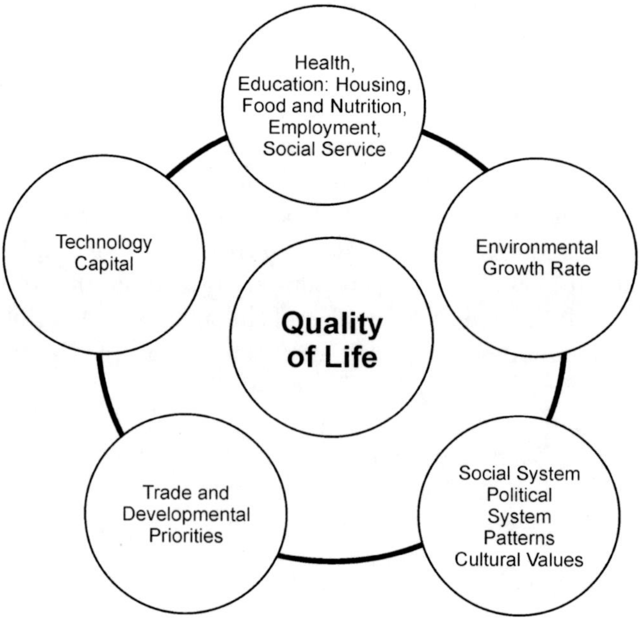

How to Impart Population Education

There are at least two main components of teaching population education – content and method. The way in which children learn about population may be just as important as what they learn about it. It is thought that since the area of population education is by its very nature problem oriented and value laden, the methods of enquiry and other student managed methods are more appropriate. A programme that helps children learn how to learn, how to investigate and how to act on problems will have a greater impact on their attitudes and beliefs than a teacher led approach, where knowledge and data are poured into them, without any need for them to use their intellect.

Teachers habitually use the same approach for practically all sorts of training objectives, in all kinds of learning situations, and with all types of audiences. Persuading the electronic media, especially radio, to increase programming on population issues is one of the tasks facing planners during 21st century. Radio, in fact, could be used far more effectively than it is. It has been estimated that there are more than 1.9 billion radios in the world – one for every three people. Radio programme are relatively inexpensive to produce, compared to film or television, and radio does not require expensive hardware. Listening to the radio is convenient; it is entertaining and people can listen while they work.

Sensitive television and radio programmes, which treat population and family planning topics in a no-nonsense fashion, can reach millions of people. Even the poorest, illiterate farmer can listen to a village radio set or watch television. India, the Philippines and the Republic of Korea were among the first countries to establish strong national family planning policies and their government owned radio and television stations have long been employed on behalf of their national population programmes.

Creating Awareness about Population Education

What should parents or teachers know about sex education? Fortunately, there are some definite yet simple answers emerging in this field, on which there is complete agreement. In the first place, it is now well established that children show an interest in sexual matters very early on. However, this interest is not a sexual interest in the adult sense. In the early years, information about such matters does not have the personal sexual meaning that adults experience. The curiosity of children about sexual differences arises normally as they become aware of their bodies and of bodily functions. The best way to deal with this curiosity is with truthful answers to the questions children ask. The answers should be given in simple, easily understood language, in a matter of fact manner without shame or embarrassment. It does not take an expert to answer the questions of children. Any adult knows all he needs to know to answer children honestly.

A range of methodologies are given below for teaching population education, and it is up to the teachers to select and use them effectively.

Lectures and lecture discussions: Student seminars, group discussions, panel discussions, debates, along with fieldwork and surveys, using questionnaires and interviews

Case studies: This method is especially effective in the study of personal and family relations and child development, and in group discussions. Case studies may be used as a basis for role playing – the spontaneous enactment or dramatization of a situation. The action comes from the students' creative use of their own feelings and imagination. It offers an excellent means of bringing emotional problems out into the open. Unlike in plays, no script, no memorization and no rehearsals are needed for role playing.

Plays and skits: A script is prepared and then presented in the form of a skit or a short play. Unlike in role play, the skit has to be memorized and rehearsed.

Value clarification strategies: The goal of this method is to enable learners to explore the connection between the subject matter and their own feelings, attitudes and behaviour. A number of value clarification models have been evolved, which are used widely.

Brainstorming: This is a technique used in solving various kinds of problems. It lists all the ideas regarding the solution of problem, without evaluating or judging them in any way.

Buzz sessions: This is an effective technique for increasing individual discussions.

Use of springboards: Springboards are thought provoking material on a topic, which motivate students into conducting an inquiry on the subject. Statements that present controversial, opposing or incompatible positions form excellent springboards.

Films, film strips and other audiovisual aids.

Self-learning: There are at least two ways in which self-learning can be conducted: (i) self-study and self-reflection on the issues contained in the self-study module, and (ii) directed self-study under the guidance of a module manager followed by group discussions. In the latter, the trainer may act as the manager.

Television has been used increasingly to inform the public about population and family planning issues. Some 20 countries have launched their own television programmes, usually in the form of educational spots or mini-plays, to promote reproductive health and family planning.

Experience has shown that the most effective way to increase public awareness of population and health related issues is to launch multimedia campaigns, employing television, radio, newspapers, magazines and specially prepared information booklets.

A well coordinated, comprehensive national strategy can reach millions of people. As discussed above, there are several approaches for teaching this essential subject. The ordinary classroom approach cannot develop the desired attitudes and beliefs with regard to population behaviour. Different approaches have to be tried and compared with the commonly adopted classroom approach.

Conclusion and Suggestions

Population education requires support from both policy makers and the community if it is to become a full-fledged part of the education system. With such support, population education can provide opportunities for learning about appropriate population issues throughout the life cycle of a human being, from the pre-school age to old age. The types of content provided will, of course, vary according to the setting and the life stages of the learners. Population education is a need today, not only for countries like India, but also all the world. To fulfil the population education target, we have to take steps such as:

- Extend the coverage of formal and non-formal population education programmes.
- Strengthen human resources.
- Ensure that project activities correspond with the problems to be solved.
- Be sensitive to cultural norms and values and differences in the gender perceptions of population education.

Population education is a new area and no model exists which can be adopted to suit the conditions prevailing in our country. We have to tread new ground, keeping in view our cultural background and present needs and future aspirations. The essence of the programme should be to give learners an insight into the totality of the issues connected with population, including the nature, causes, determinants and consequences of population growth, both at the micro and macro levels; the nature and dynamics of the reproductive process; and, finally, the possibilities of planning family size and population growth. Hopefully, the acquisition of such insights will develop understanding and attitudes that contribute positively to rational decision making, both at the individual and society level, when occasion for such decision making arises.

To quote Stephen Viederman, "the aims of education are to increase awareness and hopefully to help us achieve wisdom in the conduct of our lives, both as individuals and collectively. These aims are shared by the new field to be called population awareness education. Population education, as the result of the knowledge and understanding achieved through education, helps people make responsible decisions concerning their own reproductive behaviour. The key concept is responsible decision making, which involves knowledge and understanding of the consequences of one's own actions. This is the beginning of wisdom and represents the moral and ethical purpose of population education".

Bibliography

Arora, P. 2006. *Shalaoman Sex nu Shikshan*. Shet & Co., Mumbai.

Jain, N. 1986. Behavioural Dimensions of Population Education and Sex Education. Sociology Ph.D. dissertation, Panjab University.

Mascarenhas, M.M. 1982. *Population Education for Quality of Life*. Oxford University Press, New Delhi.

Mathur, V.S. 1996. *Some Thoughts on Population Education*. Aggarwal Prakashan, Delhi.

Negi, B.S. 2001. *Introduction of Adolescent Education in School Curriculum*. Kaniskha Publishers, New Delhi.

Prakasam, C.P. and Raju, S.S. 2006. *Adolescents' Reproductive Health Perspectives*. B.R. Publishing Corp., Delhi.

Rajani, R. 2000. *Reproductive and Sexual Health for Adolescents: Needs Assessment*. Discovery Publishing House, New Delhi.

Reddy, I.V. 1983. *Psychological Foundation of Education*. Veni Publishers, Tirupati.

Ruhela, S.P. and Husain, A. 2002. *Sex Education in India in the 21st Century*. Indian Publishers Distributors, New Delhi.

Weinberg, C. 1988. *Education and Social Problems*. The Free Press, New York.

4 Health Education

Health education, which is an amalgam of health and education, reflects the attributes of each and is committed to democratic learning processes, human dignity and community value systems. Health education can be defined as the art of applying social and health sciences to facilitate the development of healthy lifestyles and behaviour among people. Information, communication, motivation and media are essential and integral components of health education.

Health education involves multidisciplinary teamwork in planning educational strategies, in designing multimedia campaigns, in the effective use of electronic and mass media, and in folk communication activities. It is the art of working with people of various backgrounds to satisfy their needs by their own action and by mobilizing the resources of other sectors. Its main function is to create appropriate educational opportunities in varying environments for people to make their own enlightened decisions and act upon them. For this purpose, it uses the home, market and meeting place (community health education), school (school/student health education) and workplace (industrial health education) and hospital (patient education), and employs methods and medical strategies suitable to the target groups and their problems. This type of learning is as complex as it is time consuming, but when practised with sincerity and careful planning, it yields the desired results, as has been demonstrated repeatedly in many rural and urban areas of India.

Health education also includes sanitation education, population education, HIV/AIDS education, cancer education, mental health education, etc., which draw upon the concepts and principal techniques of learning processes developed in the fields of psychology, anthropology, sociology and other social sciences.

Health education is an abstract term that means different things to different people. To some, it is public relations aimed at publicizing the activities of health departments and winning public goodwill. Some consider it synonymous with propaganda. Many equate it with transmission of information about health and diseases from experts to lay clients. For others, there is no difference between health education and mass campaigns. These different perceptions are attributable both to the historical development of health education and our understanding of the learning process. Whatever those perceptions may be, the following understanding of the meaning of the term, 'health education', will be useful:

1. Health education, like general education, is concerned with changes in the knowledge, feelings and behaviour of people. This definition implies that health education has knowledge, attitude and behaviour components.
2. Health education is the translation of what is known about health into desirable individual, family and community behaviour patterns by means of the educational process. This statement implies that health education aims at individual, family and community behaviour and their interaction patterns.
3. Health education is a process leading to programmed planning, utilizing available resources, modifying health behaviour, breaking down barriers of ignorance, prejudice and misconception after an intelligent and thoughtful consideration of the relevant health knowledge.
4. Health education is the development of individual, group, institutional, community and systematic strategies to improve health knowledge, attitudes, skills and behaviour.

The World Health Organization (WHO), in its constitution, defines that health is a state of complete physical, mental and social well-being and not merely the absence of disease or infirmity. Creating a healthy world that meets this definition demands the concentrated efforts of all because health is considered a fundamental right of all human beings. Today, people live in a highly complex industrial society and, as such, the technological complexities of this society are reflected in their daily life. Modern science is bringing to people knowledge and devices that can make their life safer and healthier.

What is Education?

Education is future-oriented – it is about development and growth even when we are studying the past. As we have stressed, much thinking is commonplace – it goes on all the time, often without our being aware of it. Education takes us into the conscious world. It involves activities that are intended to stimulate thinking and foster learning. We set out to help another person to learn or to learn something ourselves (the process of self-education). Both can take place at the same time. We learn as we teach. In conversation, we learn about people and communities and also the craft of informal education.

Aims and Values of Health Education in Schools

The importance of health education has been felt in almost all the countries of the world. Medical Association and National Education Society of USA have laid the following aims and values for health education in schools:

1. Students should be given such an education that they reserve their health.
2. The students' guardians and the community should be encouraged to help in the school's health education schemes.
3. An attempt should be made to form habits in students that help them to lead healthy lives.

On the basis of the views expressed by various eminent educationists and scholars, we can say that the following should be the aims of health education programmes in schools:

1. Students should be taught the rules for the preservation and development of their physical, mental and emotional health.
2. They should be taught the causes and measures of various diseases and ailments.
3. They should be taught the rules of hygiene and encouraged to practise them in daily life.

4. Good habits should be developed in the students and they should be taught the ways of healthy living.
5. The cooperation of the community and the students' guardians should be sought in running health education programmes.
6. Health education programmes should be comprehensive and elaborate. This will help future generations to grow strong and healthy.

Health education also aims at bringing scientific knowledge to people so that they can use such knowledge for the betterment of their own health as well of the people or community in which they live. Health education is necessary because it is well known that:

1. Health cannot be thrust on people, but must be acquired through their own efforts.
2. Ignorance, prejudices and many social and cultural factors interact with health. Hence, education is needed to replace ignorance with knowledge, remove prejudices and bring about changes in belief and attitudes in a direction favourable to good health.

Importance of Health Education

It is said that a sound mind lives in a sound body. This saying clearly brings to light the importance of the health of the physical body. If the body is healthy, the mind will also be healthy. In the world of education, this has added importance: Education cannot be acquired without a proper frame of mind. A proper frame of mind cannot be achieved without proper health. Thus, it is evident that social, community and personal life cannot be successful unless there is physical health.

Scope of Health Education

Health education is a rather vast term. It includes food and its importance in the development of the body. It looks at abnormal conditions and their bad effect on health. It encompasses bad habits and their negative influence on the physical and mental health of individuals. The purpose of health education is to positively influence the health behaviour of individuals and communities as well as the living and working conditions that influence their health.

It is becoming increasingly clear, however, that not being really ill is not the same as being really well Although it is true that decreasing death rates and increasing life expectancy indicate better community health in general terms, it does not provide an accurate enough picture. As a result of improved sanitary conditions, people may live longer and enjoy a rich life of abundant vigour, serenity and joy. But equally, today, people have become so used to a state of sub-health that they do not recognize it as less than perfect. Minor disorders, such as digestive troubles, constipation, varicose veins, neuralgia, anaemia and defects of the eyes, ears and teeth, are passively accepted as one's lot in life. The average level of health has come to be regarded as optimal, but we cannot be completely satisfied until the average is the optimal. We have added years to life; what is now needed is that we add life to the years.

One difficulty about this concept of 'positive health' is that while we have morbidity statistics which give a picture of the degree of illness of a community, we have as yet no means of measuring the community's degree of health and vigour. Even to measure the degree of health of an individual in any terms other than the absence of defects and disease is difficult, but while perfect health cannot be easily defined, healthy people have certain characteristics that may be fairly readily recognized. They have a sense of general fitness and of competence and joy in bodily movement; they find exercise enjoyable; relaxation and sleep come easily when they are tired; they have hearty appetites and easy elimination; in most cases, their height and weight do not vary widely from the normal; they are able to adjust themselves rapidly to variations in climatic and other environmental conditions; their intelligence is adequate to the needs of daily life and their mental processes go on smoothly and efficiently; they are generally happy, self-confident and cooperative; they are not unduly troubled by worries, fears or other emotional difficulties; and they rarely wonder whether or not they are healthy. People without these or similar characteristics cannot be said to be really healthy even if they have no aches or pains serious enough to send them to a doctor.

The Need to Consider Local Conditions and Needs

The wealth or poverty of a community, its standard of education, home circumstances and customs vary greatly in different localities. These differences must influence the local approach to health education if the subject is to be taught realistically.

Special attention should be paid to local customs and practices likely to affect health, and it will be necessary to treat these cautiously, even if their effect on health is bad. Traditional customs are not likely to be removed by the community at a moment's notice, and any attempt to bring this about may well arouse the opposition of parents and create confusion in the minds of the pupils.

On the other hand, there are some undesirable practices such as the insanitary disposal of excrement, rubbish and other waste matter, the desultory care of infants, etc., which are merely the result of ignorance or laziness. These matters can be dealt with more directly in health education and quicker results can be expected. In studying the local situation, the cooperation and, if possible, the active assistance of the students' parents should be sought as well as that of other agencies undertaking health education; of these, the most important is the staff of the local health centre.

Again for local reasons, such as climate differences between states and even districts, in the nature and distribution of disease, choice and local availability of food, house building materials and drainage problems, the school authorities should take the help of the local department, which is concerned with the community development programme. The curriculum can then be prepared to suit the conditions of the district and the needs of the community.

Content Areas of Health Education

There is considerable knowledge and information that may be taught in health education. While much of this is available in literature that is available in such forms as textbooks, resource books, pamphlets and promotional material, it is important that the content of the specific course be selected with care. At the present time, there is little uniformity in the content of health education courses being taught in schools throughout the country.

Health knowledge is important and can be justified only as the pupils apply it to their own lives and the lives of the individuals around them. There are several ways in which this vital information may be obtained. First, the interest and needs of the target students may be determined through an analysis of health records, which every school should keep in a cumulative manner and which contain such valuable information as the result of health appraisals and health counselling. Second, teachers' observations offer some indication of interest, desires and health problems. Third, tests of knowledge, attitudes and habits uncover superstitions and other health problems, together with the accuracy of the health knowledge possessed by the students. Fourth, conferences with parents, teachers and pupils reveal many health interests and needs. Fifth, a student interest survey will indicate interest in the field of health, as the students themselves see them. Sixth, a study of the current literature concerned with scientific information in the field of health is essential. Finally, a study of the health of the community is imperative in order to tailor the course to the local setting, with its own specific industrial, housing, sanitation, water supply and other problems.

These are the basic needs for everyday living:

1. Proper building materials
2. Proper use and care of the body
3. Ego preservation and enhancement
4. Protection against or control of disease producing germs
5. Protection from excessive forces
6. Food and nutrition
7. Care of the ears, eyes, teeth and mouth, skin, scalp and hair
8. Clothing
9. Posture
10. Play
11. Fresh air and sunshine
12. Sleep, rest and relaxation
13. Healthy home, school and community
14. Prevention of disease
15. Temperance
16. Healthy personality
17. Safety

The Government of India has developed an excellent syllabus in health education for schools. In addition to covering the considerable introductory material on the importance of health in school programmes, it contains the following topics as well:

1. Maintaining and improving mental health
2. Developing wholesome life relationships
3. Communicable diseases and sanitation
4. Community health
5. Personal health, which includes the following resource units:
   (a) Nutrition education
   (b) Dental health
   (c) Rest, work, relaxation
   (d) Eyes, ears, nose, throat
   (e) Heart and circulation
   (f) Alcohol education
   (g) Narcotics education
   (h) Personal cleanliness and grooming
   (i) Posture education, including care of the feet
   (j) Cancer education
6. First aid
7. HIV/AIDS awareness.

Biology curricula in schools still emphasize content such as morphology and anatomy. An analysis of the content might suggest that there is much relevant to health, but it follows a strictly logical sequence with little application to real life situations. The information within the logical structure is to be memorized as is other information in science. It is not included with the main purpose of improving the health of the learners.

The people who should be informed of the life cycle, its effects on human health, and the suffering and lack of productivity that it causes are schoolchildren. Yet, in biology teaching, is merely presented as a 'flat worm' in the sequence of invertebrate orders, while its relationship to human health is shyly presented as a secondary issue. If curriculum planners realize the gravity of such a parasite and how much damage it causes to human health and to the economy of the country, they should change the emphasis of presentation from 'just another worm' to a menace that does so much damage and can be controlled through many channels, the most effective of which is education.

Another example is how the human body system is explained to schoolchildren. This happens mainly in Classes 7–9. The structure of the system is presented thoroughly with anatomical details. But there is almost no reference to hygiene of the human body, which is of such importance to the nation's health. Although there are references in the syllabus to care of the human body, nutrition, parasites and bacteria, and pollution, these are presented as secondary issues. No major health concepts have been clearly defined or developed through the years of study,

Young people need to know certain biological facts of life at certain ages in order to meet and solve the problems that they will face. Facts about reproduction, family life, growth and development, diseases and similar issues are rarely mentioned in biology courses. Developing proper health skills, habits and attitudes is not one of the objectives of biology, and teaching skills and attitudes related to nutrition, sanitation and pollution control, protection against contagious diseases, and child care are rarely mentioned. Unfortunately, students do not usually learn proper skills and habits from their families or their communities. This makes it vital that they are helped to develop these through the school curriculum. Teachers can promote respect and understanding of the medical services in the community. The role of biology teachers in giving guidance is too often overlooked. In most cases, students do not dare to ask their teachers about the problems that are causing them anxieties in their lives. Questions about sex, family life, and growth and development are among the important questions that biology teachers should answer frankly and scientifically.

Role of the Family

Cleanliness is undoubtedly an acquired taste, but it is not merely an aesthetic value. Above all, it is a sanitary safeguard, the importance of which has been learnt through hard experience. In other words, to be clean is in a large measure to be safe from infectious diseases.

Cleanliness applies not only to people, but also to their personal environment. Environmental cleanliness is a highly important factor in sanitation. This is especially true when food is related to the idea of cleanliness. Any suggestion of dirt connected with food or food stuff, including dirty cooking vessels, brings about an almost universal dissatisfaction and disgust.

It is to biological cleanliness or freedom from bacteria that health owes its greatest debt. As living microbes are the causes of disease, freedom from these means freedom from disease. A clean personal environment has an equally great hygienic value. No one should use a common drinking cup. Contaminated water and infected milk should be excluded, or rendered clean and free from bacteria by boiling before use. Purification by cooking is one of the greatest sanitary advances ever made by man and is the only means of rendering food safe for consumption.

If the lessons of cleanliness that children learn at home are reinforced at school, they leave a deep impression that lasts through their lives. As children learn many things at home consciously or unconsciously, the family plays an important role in imparting health education.

Personal cleanliness is as important as the cleanliness of the house, street and places of resort. The public should be convinced of the usefulness of clean surroundings. This can be accomplished by proper instruction of children and adults in the technical knowhow of cleanliness based upon proper knowledge, and this knowledge should be translated into habits. An important preventive measure is the provision of health education for parents. Modern parents must be aware of facts regarding child development and the physical, emotional and social needs of children, prevention of illness, care of sick children, protection from common dangers, and promoting the greatest possible potential development of the intellect by education, as well as the skills in applying them. They should be aware of the medical and social services that are available in their community.

Village Sanitation

Modern notions of sanitation are quite unknown to Indians, especially those living in rural areas. Village houses are usually built of mud or bricks, with roofs of palm thatching or country tiles. They stand in rows and are ill-ventilated, there being few or no windows. The rooms, especially in the interior of the house, where the women and children sleep and work, are generally dark and unventilated. The houses are too close to each other and the lanes too narrow to allow free air and sunlight. Often, there are cattle sheds in the front of the house. All household sewage flows into the lanes.

Here are some measures that could improve the sanitation in villages:

1. Provision of a protected water supply.
2. Efficient drainage.
3. Prompt removal of refuse and excreta from human habitations.

Role of Voluntary Agencies

Voluntary organizations have a vital role to play in almost all spheres of political, economic and social reforms. In a developing country where welfare measures are still embryonic, voluntary organizations fulfil a fundamental need by endeavouring to ameliorate the conditions of the disadvantaged by supplementing and complementing existing services, by being the instruments of change, and by serving as catalysts for community action, which, ultimately, is the best way of achieving progress in any society. Voluntary agencies can help in designing the format of curricula by identifying the availability of local resources, checking on the health needs of the people, and analysing the methodology of instruction most suitable to the local environment.

In recent years, with Central Government financial support becoming more generous, public health agencies, too, are extending their services to communities. Today, many state departments of health employ health education specialists, who devote themselves entirely to health education. Several state departments of education have also recognized the importance of health education and their respective states have provided funds for the development of a staff to disseminate such education. When state government agencies are well supplied with Central Government funds, their cooperation is easy. The test of cooperation between the state departments of education and health will arise when Central Government funds are cut off. The department of education needs factual data and scientific guidance in many areas from the department of health and the department of health needs teaching methods and techniques for presenting scientific material to varied groups from the department of education. The administrative machinery for cooperation at the state level might well be an interdepartmental committee with representation from the education, health, welfare and other interested departments, all working together to solve health problems.

Voluntary health associations (VHAs) link more than 4,000 health care institutions and grass roots community health programmes spread across the country. VHAs can have communications units that publish health education material, community health and development units that conduct training programmes, information units that maintain health, development and family welfare related information, and women's health and drugs units. VHAs and other special educational institutions working in the field of adult education can encourage the development of curricula and provide financial assistance for the purpose. University departments of continuing and adult education, teachers' training colleges and state resource centres can provide useful data. At the national level, the Directorate of Adult Education, the Indian Adult Education Association and other national specialized agencies can organize workshops for key personnel engaged in curriculum construction with a view to providing general guidelines and orientation. They can fill the void, tackle issues and deal with needs that others may not even recognize or are unable or unwilling to face. Many of them are involved in training, education and counselling services, which involve sensitizing and motivating the community to participate actively in related activities, development of information, education and communication (IEC) materials, etc.

VHAs can arrange capacity building workshops for state partners called Building Health Promoting Schools and Communities. The agenda of the workshops can be innovative programmes and providing the participants with exposure to their counterparts in other states in order to enable them to improve their programmes and share their views, experiences and challenges. Action research and evaluative studies can be undertaken by a number of agencies and institutions, both governmental and non-governmental. Mention may be made in this connection of the programme evaluation organization of the Planning Commission, university departments of education and allied subjects, state resource centres, and specialized agencies, including voluntary organizations of repute in the field of adult health education.

Health Education in Relation to Community and School Health Programmes

It has already been established that health education is one part of the total school health programme. It is usual for the educational component of the total programme to be the most obvious and the part most people think about, especially those involved in the preparation of the relationship of the health education component to other aspects of the school health programme. So, it is fitting to point out ways in which health education relates to school health services, the school health environment and the community health programme.

There are different ways in which these two aspects of the total school health programme connect with each other:

1. Classroom discussions before and/or after health service activities can be educational.
2. Classroom discussions about health service activities can help foster more positive feelings about the activities and relationships with health service personnel.
3. Health service personnel may have the expertise to contribute to the health education curriculum and/or teaching.
4. Health services personnel are often in a position to provide support for educational programmes.
5. Health services results can provide case studies or other statistical evidence to help in health education.
6. Health educators, through observations, can notice students who need the health services.

The very fact that health services are provided establishes teaching opportunities. For example, elementary school students may be very interested in learning about vision just before or after they have had their vision tested. Simple height and weight statistics can lead to interesting discussions about the broad topic of growth and development. Since students have just been subjected to some types of health services, their questions will take on significance for them that might not be apparent at any other time. Some individuals have negative feelings about health services and personnel. If the health services associated with the school are well conducted, the service providers can help educate the students about the reasons for the need of the services as well as remove some of the negative feelings that might exist about health personnel. Classroom discussions can lead to greater understanding of the roles of the personnel and the goals of the health services.

All individuals involved in health services must have a high degree of expertise in some areas of total health in order to be effective in providing the services. This expertise may be useful in health education programmes. While these individuals are probably extremely busy, they should not be overlooked as potential human resources by those planning the educational component. It is likely that human resources have practical information that is almost impossible to find in any textbook. Even if health services personnel do not have much time to contribute directly to educational programmes, their understanding of the programmes is essential since they are probable sources of support for the programme. People who provide health services are often regarded as experts in health, though this does not necessarily mean that they are experts in the total area of health. But since they are often thought of as experts, their support of educational endeavours can be of great benefit. It may only be necessary to have a health services person say a few positive words about the need for better health education. Administrators and the community in general may be much more likely to support health education if they know the health services personnel are also supporting it.

Health educators should be alert for information from health services publications that might relate to educational experiences. For example, the analysis of case studies about a particular health problem might lead to consideration of such questions as: How was the problem detected? Why was it important to detect the problem?

What might have happened if the problem was not detected? What personal health behaviour might have influenced the health problem? The possibilities are endless when individual differences and environmental influences are added to the list of possible considerations related to particular health problems. Actual health service examples can make certain aspects of education seem more realistic, up to date and to the point.

The final connection between health education and health services to be mentioned here is the detective role of health educators. Teachers' observations can be an important source for referral of students who may be in need of particular health services. Certain students may seem to experience difficulty in hearing, seeing or speaking. The problem could be something less obvious, such as a change of temperament or work habits. But these are symptoms that educators might notice. Thus, the observations of educators can be very helpful to students and the health services in detecting potential problems early and can be of great assistance to the school health services programme.

Health Education as Lifelong Education

Health education has become a part of lifelong education. As health education is required for almost everyone in society and it is required in a continuous manner, it is wrong to assume that health education is required for only formal education. It is true that even people who are otherwise highly educated may not know enough about health matters, and if they do know, their behaviour may be not be fully conducive to good health. For example, the ill effects of overeating, smoking and drinking alcohol may be well known to well educated people, but they may continue to do these in their daily lives.

It can be appreciated that health education is needed for all ages, sexes, classes of community, whether rich or poor, literate or illiterate, and in all parts of the world. Even in the developed countries, health education becomes important because of the changing conditions of life. Science helps us discover many new aspects about diseases and health, which is why health education is a never ending process.

Thus, health education has to do with knowing the health needs of a community and acting to fulfil those needs. It is a process in which people are helped to learn what is good for themselves and their health and to adopt patterns of behaviour that will ensure normal health. This process of health education implies that people should be able to follow healthful ways of living voluntarily, after having understood the need for such behaviour.

Health education is the joint responsibility of both homes and schools. Neither schools nor homes, in isolation, can help in the satisfactory health development of children. Health education must be accepted by the administrative authorities of the school as an essential part of the education programme if it is to be successful. Effective health education demands the understanding, sympathy, cooperation and support of health specialists, doctors, nurses, dentists, nutritionists and physical educationists, who are expected to understand, contribute to and cooperate in health training programmes.

Bibliography

Adiseshia, M. 1982. 'Adult Education and Urban Poor', in *Teacher Today*, January.

Datta, S.C. 1983. 'Education for All: An Alternative Strategy', in *Indian Journal of Adult Education (IJAE)*, Vol. 44, No. 12.

Kundu, C.L. 1978. *Adult Education*. Sterling Publishers, New Delhi.

Manelkar, R.K. 1997. *A Textbook of Community Health for Nurses*. Vora Medical Publications, Mumbai.

Ministry of Education and Social Welfare. 1999. Training of Adult Education Functionaries. New Delhi.

Ministry of Health and Family Welfare. 1978. Handbook on PNDT Act., New Delhi.

Mishra, R.C. 2005. *HIV/AIDS Education*. A.P.H. Publishing Corp., New Delhi.

National AIDS Control Organization. 1994. AIDS Education: A Training Package. National Council for Educational Research and Training and NACO, Delhi, pp. 66–71.

World Health Organization. 1994. *Bench Aids for the Diagnosis of Intestinal Parasites*. WHO, Geneva.

World Health Organization. 2002. *Reducing Risks, Promoting Healthy Life*. WHO, Geneva.

Yadav, C.P. 2007. *Encyclopaedia of HIV/AIDS, Problems and Control*. Anmol Publications, New Delhi.

5 Teaching Methods for Health Education

Before understanding the different teaching methods that can be used in health education programmes, it is necessary to develop an understanding of what is health education. Through the years, there have been a variety of definitions of health education, just as there have been a variety of definitions of health itself. As definitions of health were accepted within programmes, a certain style of health education would follow logically. For example, if health were defined as the absence of disease, then the health education programme would centre upon disease prevention. Sometimes, health was considered in terms of statistical relationships, such as how many people have a certain characteristic, in an attempt to improve the statistical situation.

In order to appreciate the total scope of health education today, it is necessary to accept a broad based definition of health. Health encompasses all phases of living, including the psychological, sociological, biological and spiritual. Even though these characteristics are listed separately, in reality, they exist together and intermingle in order to result in a state of health. It is this kind of health that contemporary health education focuses upon.

Health education strategies provide needed approaches to bridging the gap between scientific discoveries and their application in everyday healthful living. Within many other disciplines, knowledge is discovered every day, which may relate to the health of people. Health education utilizes this wealth of information and, through appropriate teaching strategies, attempts to integrate this knowledge into people's daily living patterns. Knowledge may be nice to know, but it must find its way into common understanding and use before it is of any practical value.

Health education contributes to the total education of individuals by providing meaningful experiences that can positively influence health behaviour. The proof of the success of health education lies in the healthier practices adopted by people over the years. It is easy to show that health education has a positive effect upon health knowledge, but the challenge of influencing health behaviour over a long period of time remains the real test.

Health education is most appropriately engaged in by professionally prepared health educators. There is such a vast amount of health knowledge and it takes a skilful person to attempt to influence people' health behaviour, so it is crucial that professionals trained as health educators perform the bulk of health education in today's times.

Aubrey called health education the 'neglected child of the schools' and indicated that at least six factors have contributed to poor health education programmes:

1. *Inadequate training of teachers during college preparation:* This can apply to all teachers, but especially to those being prepared to teach in the elementary grades and those desiring to teach full time health education. If their own training is not adequate or appropriate, it is not surprising teachers are unable to teach properly.
2. *Lack of enforcement of mandatory state regulations concerning the teaching of health:* If the existing regulations are not enforced, often, there are inadequate funds for the personnel and for programme materials. It is also easy in those circumstances for administrators and teachers to 'forget about' teaching health.
3. *Resistance and apathy of teachers:* Teachers may not care about teaching health because they may feel uneasy with some of the topics covered under it. They may not feel that health education is important because they have only seen 'rainy day' classes or poor programmes themselves. Yet, they are also busy teaching the material within their own disciplines.

4. *Indifference and low priority of health among school administrators:* Administrators may be fearful of strong parental reactions to the inclusion of some of the more 'sensitive' health topics. It may be easier to do nothing since regulations are often not enforced and little outside pressure may exist.
5. *Difficulties in building student interest and involvement:* This situation is easy to understand if often used health textbooks and health education methods are examined. The books tend to be outdated, the classes too large, and the emphasis may be upon memory work and not enough on dealing with topics of interest and importance.
6. *Parental resistance and indifference:* Since many parents have been through poor health education programmes themselves, it is difficult for many of them to understand the reasons for the programme for their children or what should be within it. They may also be fearful of some of the topics they hear about in health education.

As we all know, education has many meanings. An analysis of the word reveals a number of commonly employed definitive names. There are those who would confine education to the teaching and learning process. Some would define it as the process of helping the maturing individual to make the transition smoothly into the life and culture of the group. Others would restrict the concept still further to the conscious and purposeful control of learning by the more experienced members of society. Still others would limit education to the work of certain special agencies, such as the tutor and the school, which are presumably devoted exclusively to the twofold task of teaching and learning. If education is regarded primarily as the gradual, smooth induction of the maturing individual into the life and culture of the group, and if the group is broadly conceived to include the dead as well as the living, then this process is clearly essential to both the renewal and the growth of human society. In its absence, the achievement of society would be limited by the powers and to the experiences of individuals, and what is known as culture could not develop.

Education is well recognized as a continuous learning process, which begins with the birth of the child and persists through its life. Accordingly, a system of public education is no longer limited to the provision of elementary and secondary education, but consists of schools and institutions as varied as the needs of the individuals that make up a community. The meaning, then, of the phrase, 'community health education', is a process employed in meeting the physical and mental needs of the social organization as expressed in health.

Much skill is needed in successful health education for it is never sufficient just to tell people about a special subject. If possible, those being taught should be involved. This means that successful health education depends on first learning as much as possible about the audience. Discussions and arguments are valuable and, while a teaching session should never be too long, it should help in clearing thoughts and imparting education.

There are three main methods of health education:

- Individual health education.
- Group health education.
- Mass media health education.

Individual Health Education

This is always the most effective method because most people learn quickly in this manner and the results are more lasting. It includes personal discussions between patients and doctors, nurses and health instructors, and simple demonstrations. Much individual health education can be carried out in connection with ordinary medical, nursing or social workers in the course of everyday tasks.

Group Health Education

This occurs when a small group of people – six to eight – are taught together wherever possible – in child health clinics, schools or factories. Group discussions should be promoted so that everyone plays on active part. Talks should be short – 5–10 minutes – and various visual aids, such as film strips, colour slides and 16 mm films, should be used. Group health education can be particularly useful when the individual finds it difficult to follow the health advice being given, as in the case of someone attempting to give up smoking or trying to lose weight. The group itself helps to support the individuals in these instances.

Mass Media Health Education

In this technique, the topics are presented to the whole community by means of radio, television, posters and other methods designed to keep them in the public eye. Different types of topics can be taught using this method; examples include the prevention of accidents and general diseases, immunization, nutrition and the dangers of smoking. Mass media health education is only effective if it is supported by other means, such as individual and group discussions.

Education is both science and art. It involves the question of not only what to teach, but also how to teach it. Every educational work, therefore, has its own educational method. The methods of health education are the most effective ways of executing any programme connected with it. In India, where illiteracy is a big problem, it is obvious that traditional methods such as lectures and talks would not serve the purpose fully. So, the education methods should be target oriented to make them effective.

Lectures and Talks

A lecture series is a series of presentations given by a lecturer over a period, like one per day, one per week or one per month. Quite often, these lectures are related to a specific topic and are delivered by outside experts or speakers who provide the information to a target group.

Lectures can be organized by community workers and expert talks can be given by doctors. The topic can be related to an ongoing problem in the community; for example, if there are water and sanitation problems, possible topics for lectures and talks could be gastroenteritis, cholera, malaria and typhoid. The ultimate object is to promote better understanding of the issues and to facilitate a meaningful dialogue between learned experts and those directly concerned with the problem. While giving the lecture, the expert can use illustrations, pictures and diagrams for better clarity, as, for example, for decreased menstrual flow, excessive white discharge, ulceration of the mouth of the uterus, etc.

Advantages

- More content can be included.
- It is quite simple for the experts.

Disadvantages

- One needs to work hard to develop the lecture.
- It is a time consuming method.
- It can become boring, as a result of which the listeners may lose their attention.

Demonstrations

Demonstrations are a method of showing how something works, what it is composed of and why it is important. People become involved in demonstrations because they are looking at a specific thing which holds their attention. Demonstrations can be used to show clean methods of food preparation, new techniques of sanitation, how to preserve food, and so on. Demonstrations can be given by teachers, outside experts or students. It is a valuable activity for villagers because it makes them participate in the process of communication. Demonstrations of cheap and nutritious meals can be a very effective way of imparting health education. Similarly, mothers can be taught how to care for their babies using demonstrations of the infants' weight and length, using standard methods.

Objectives

Demonstrations are used to provide awareness regarding improved practices and how one practice is superior to another, as, for example, how solar energy is more useful than electronic energy.

- They bring research to the doors of the users.
- They show the actual process to the learners, which makes for clear understanding.

- They are used as a vital media for communication determination and diffusion of information.
- They uphold the principles of seeing is believing and learning by doing.

Advantages

- Demonstrations attract and hold the attention and arouse the learners' interest.
- They present the subject matter in a way that can be understood easily.
- They convince those who might otherwise doubt that a thing could be done or that they themselves could do it.
- The demonstration method is objective and concrete.
- Demonstrations permit the teaching of theory along with practice.

Disadvantages

- Good demonstrations are not easy.
- The demonstration method is restricted to only certain kinds of teaching situations.
- The result type of demonstrations may take considerable time and be rather expensive.
- Demonstrations may require a large amount of preliminary preparation.

Group Discussions

Group discussions are held with small groups of two – 10 people, though there could be larger groups, too.

- A small group is an ideal unit for teaching because it encourages the involvement of the learners in the learning process.
- It permits actions, reactions and interactions between the learners and the teacher, as well as among the learners.
- It allows the rearrangement of physical facilities – such as the sitting patterns and placing of teaching aids – if needed.

- It is suitable or appropriate for individualized learning, especially for problem solving decision making and analysing a situation or concept.
- It helps in galvanizing efforts by the formation of voluntary health groups through monthly health and immunization days and improved reach and quality of health services by linkages with health providers.

Methods of Discussion for Small Groups

Each method of presentation will require discussion before, during and after the presentation of the subject matter or content. No particular method of discussion can be recommended for small groups, in isolation of the method of presentation. Both the presentation and discussion should go hand in hand.

Small group discussions are a good method because all the learners in the group can participate, there is more time available, and group conclusions can be arrived at. A common theme or topic, reassigned to the group, with sources of data located, will yield good results from group discussions. For example, sessions on HIV/AIDS and puzzles and quizzes on HIV/AIDS, followed by focus group discussions can help in imparting sound health education. Awareness about HIV/AIDS leads to a healthy attitude to sexuality and to the development of a healthy lifestyle, which reduces the risk of HIV/AIDS among adolescents. It provides knowledge and life skills to shape the adolescents of today as healthy individuals of the future.

Focus Group Discussions

This method permits in-depth discussions in small groups. Focus group discussions are guided by the expert, but the learners talk freely and spontaneously on the topics selected by the group. A family, which is a homogenous small group, which is also well prepared, can produce a rich stock of the data necessary for in-depth discussions, as, for example, on reproductive health.

Limitations and Precautions for Small Groups

- The expert plays the additional role of promoting individualized learning because individual learning experiences are provided to all the learners in the group.
- If the learners do not or cannot develop the skills to discuss, present, question and recap, the expert is forced to be a lecturer, rather than a director or facilitator of learning.
- With poor reading habits and low motivation on the part of the learners, small groups can be boring. Such groups may also be too informal to create a somewhat controlled/structured environment to promote learning.
- The learners can see the expert and he, in turn, can get frequent feedback from them. This is an advantage to both the expert and the learners. Focus group discussions can deal with topics such as reproductive health, family planning, and solid and liquid waste management. In fact, it can cover any topic that poses a common problem for the community and about which all the members of the community feel equally concerned.
- It helps in the promotion of health education, not only for the beneficiaries in the community who have become conscious and who have recognized their role in protecting the health and safety of their families, but for the community as a whole.

Plays

This method of teaching involves the use of dialogue and action to interpret situations and events. It differs from role play in that it usually involves a longer period of time and uses a fully developed plot. Dramatic skits are rehearsed in advance and usually play more heavily on the emotions of the observers.

Objectives

- Plays offer opportunities to the performers to use their own intelligence, talent and imagination while performing on the stage.

- They help the performers make use of their imagination and come out with innovative and new results.
- The performers get a platform to showcase their emotions.
- Plays help to remove social problems and provide awareness in an interesting manner.
- They provide opportunities to communicate through actions, words, sound, rhythm, etc.

Selection of Plays

Plays should centre round the felt needs of the people of a community. For example, if the health status of a particular village is very poor and it also faces the problem of having to navigate kachcha roads, first priority should be given to conducting plays on how to improve the health status, using topics such as the ill effects of poor nutrition and frequent pregnancies on women, leading to the understanding that women's health cannot be isolated from their social status. In most of rural India, women and girls drink less milk than their husbands and sons and they eat only after the men have eaten. This usually leaves women with a limited diet, which tells us a lot about how much they are valued. Such topics can be shown easily through plays.

Planning a Play

- Care should be taken to evoke emotions in the play that most of the audience can sense themselves.
- The script should be flexible and the action as spontaneous as possible.
- The objectives should be defined clearly.
- The issue to be dramatized should be clear, meaningful and well defined.

Role Plays

Role play is the spontaneous acting out of an incident by selected members of a group to portray a human relationship problem that is common to the members of the group. Roles are usually assigned to various members of the group, who then act out the problem situation. For example, health and hygiene is a big problem in our slum communities and in rural India. Role play can be effectively used to raise awareness about the need for proper sanitation facilities, health check-ups, prevention of transmission of diseases through the proper disposal of human excreta, and about the bad effects of contamination of water and soil. This will help in improving the sanitary conditions of households and their nearby environment.

Advantages

- The method is new and novel.
- It provides for more active participation by the group members.
- It introduces the situation to both the actors and observers with a dramatic impact.
- It can arouse interest in the problem.
- It can help in clarifying the problem.

Disadvantages

- Role play is not always an appropriate method. If the situation is not suited to the use of the technique, role play is a mere waste of time.
- It requires a lot of time.
- It becomes ineffective if it runs for too long.
- It becomes useless if the topic is not related to the target group.
- It becomes ineffective when one person begins performing various roles.

Street Plays

Also called street theatre, these are plays that are performed on streets or in busy places. Street plays are a recent phenomenon. They provide a link between the highly sophisticated play and the improvised role play. In cities, they are usually performed on streets or in slums. In villages, they are performed at key places, such as prominent road crossings, the village square, or near a busy market-place or temple. Street plays usually seek to create awareness about government policies related to health and social problems. The government may pass any number of welfare measures, but they are useless unless the people get to know of them and step forward to avail of them. So, social workers started conducting programmes to pass the message on to the people. They visit certain areas and perform street plays, which informed the people of the area about the welfare measures, thereby combining learning and entertainment. Street plays can take up all kinds of developmental issues. They can also create awareness regarding health issues and their solutions. For example, anaemia, or deficiency of iron, is a highly prevalent and seemingly stubborn problem, particularly among children, adolescent girls and pregnant women in India. Street plays are very effective in communicating information about anaemia and its alleviation.

Preparing for Street Plays

Selection of the Topic

First of all, the performers should analyse the problem of the community before which they are going to perform the street play. Then they can write a script and give it an attractive name.

Selection of Characters

The characters in street plays should be decided according to skills and ability and then assigned to individual characters.

Writing the Script

The following steps should be kept in mind while writing a script:

Decide the Theme

- The message should be clear.
- Street plays should not last more than 40–45 minutes, otherwise they will become boring.

Make a Story

- Think up a story in a storytelling form that is interesting.

- Decide on the characters.
- Provide script dialogue to the characters.
- Avoid having too many characters in one play.

Practice

Perfection requires practice and performers should remain alert so that if one performer forgets a dialogue, he or the others should bridge the gap and carry on with the play. In the normal course, street plays do not require elaborate arrangements – only some open space for the performance and some clean area around for the audience.

Conducting Street Plays

- Invite the audience to join in.
- Use folk songs and bells to attract people to the performance.
- Use the local language of the target group.
- Use a friendly approach.
- The performers should have full knowledge about the issue.

Advantages

- Street plays help in solving both social and health problems.
- The performers visit the same place repeatedly, so relationships develop with the audience.
- Street plays do not require heavy budgets.
- They are closer to literary dramatic pieces.
- The actors do not need to wear specific or elaborate costumes.
- Street plays are an effective method of conveying a message to people because of the action, expression and dialogues used in them.
- They use folk songs and folk dances, so they create a feeling of belonging.
- They are an effective method of raising consciousness about health problems.

Disadvantages

- Street plays are useless if the target group fails to understand the message.
- They require a lot of planning.
- Sometimes, people take them for mere entertainment, without learning anything from them.
- They are useless if the theme is not related to the needs of the target group.
- They require prewritten scripts and plenty of practice.
- If the actors do not perform well, the message may not be effective.
- Before performing street plays, the performers need to take permission from the concerned higher authorities.

Bhavai

Bhavai is a colourful and vigorous form of folk dance-drama native to North Gujarat. In its original form, *bhavai* was a purely religious and developmental folk dance-drama, performed before the Goddess Amba, for the eradication of darkness and illusion. With the passage of time, *bhavai* has acquired many secular elements.

Bhavai has three categories – Pauranic, historical and social – and it usually presents mythological and historical romances and pokes fun at the hypocrisy of society. It uses satire as a medium. The ills of society, such as an old man marrying a young girl, wasteful expenditure on marriages and death ceremonies, or the corrupt practices of social and political leaders, are all exposed through *bhavai*.

Bhavai usually has three main characters – *nayak*, *ranglo* and *rangli*. The *nayak* is the *sutradhar* or manager. He is a singer, vocalist, narrator and director all in one. The *ranglo* is the jester or clown and the *rangli* his helpmate, who keeps him on track. The *ranglo* makes all kinds of satirical remarks.

Many health issues can be tackled through *bhavai*, as, for example, the ill effects of the use of firewood, cow dung and crop residues in household hearths on women; all these create domestic pollution and leave women vulnerable to the harmful effects of inhaling smoke over a long period, including heart disease. Carbon monoxide, which is commonly released from such fires, is a toxic gas, which reduces the haemoglobin content in blood. Continuous inhalation of carbon monoxide also leads to heart disease and impairs foetal development. Such and other similar topics on health issues can be covered effectively through the colourful *bhavai.*

Purpose

- To examine a delicate problem in human relations.
- To explore possible solutions to an emotion laden or health problem.
- To provide insights into attitudes differing sharply from those of the participants.

Seating Arrangement

- The seating arrangement should be semi-circular, with the stage in front of the audience.

Advantages

- *Bhavai* is a simple and low cost method of public communication.
- It focuses attention on a single problem at a time and learners deal with it themselves.
- It is a dramatic way of presenting a problem and stimulating discussion.
- It can provide clues to the possible solution of a health problem.

Disadvantages

- A *bhavai* can stretch too long.
- If the learners are not fully involved, it can hamper learning.
- If the objectives are not well defined and not kept in mind, it may remain a mere source of entertainment.

Campaigns

The *Oxford Dictionary* defines a campaign as an organized course of action directed towards the arousal of public interest for a particular purpose. It is an intensive act for a brief period at the proper time. It is a concentrated use of different communication methods and media around a theme for a specific period of time. It creates wide public awareness and disseminates a specific message.

Planning

- The problem with which the campaign will deal should be decided on the basis of local needs with the help of leaders and specialists.
- Once a theme is decided, a meeting should be held in the community to fix the events.
- Draw up a concrete plan highlighting the number of activities, dates and materials required.
- Decide how to involve people in the events.
- Select a period suitable to the community and announce the dates in advance.

Conducting Meetings

Meeting with popular personality, scientists, and leaders on relevant theme at public places and when people come together that is the correct time to create health awareness.

Newspaper Articles

Leaflets provide information, posters remind people of important messages through slogans or attractive visuals, and wall newspapers provide regular health information, as, for example, was done in the anti-polio campaign.

Exhibitions

Villagers are fond of going to *melas* and exhibitions. Scientific exhibitions provide a good opportunity to attract crowds and offer health education.

Advantages

- Campaigns reach many people and, thus, make health education easy.

- They provide quick results at low costs.
- They build community confidence.
- They are useful when the entire community realizes their importance.
- They need the creation of a psychological climate for the adoption of new health practices.
- They must cater to the local community as a whole.

What to Do?

- Examine local needs.
- Consult local leaders.
- Consult specialists.
- Ensure technical services and supplies.
- Select a period suitable to the community.
- Announce the dates in advance.
- Build up the enthusiasm of the people.
- Work with and through the local leaders.
- Work as per plan.
- Watch the campaign contact and find out the failures and analyse.
- Make individual contacts and find out their reactions.

Limitations

Campaigns are advantageous only when all the participants cooperate. They are not useful if the topic involves complicated technicalities.

They involve thorough preparation and close association of the concerned agencies.

They are applicable to only a few topics.

Examples of recent successful health education campaigns innovated by the Health Education, Department of Government of India are:

- Save the Girl Child
- Educating the Girl Child
- Stop Female Foeticide
- Stop the Declining Sex Ratio

- Ladka Ladki Ek Samaan (Boys and Girls are Equal)

Local campaigns can be used from time to time to encourage a certain topic, as, for example, immunization or accident prevention. Excellent results can be obtained in this way by using a community mobilization technique, whereby volunteers are asked to visit 15–20 homes to contact the occupants to cooperate in the campaign. Spectacular results have been obtained by using this method.

In conclusion, it can be said that different teaching methods, such as expert talks, demonstrations, role play, street plays and *bhavai*, can be used effectively for the promotion of health education. This holds truer for our country because India has a large number of people with no social, economic or health security and, therefore, the problem has assumed critical and devastating proportions. The different teaching methods we have discussed here, along with information, education and communication (IEC) material, can definitely achieve changes in the mindsets of people.

Health education is a process that can be considered effective when it enriches the knowledge of people and brings about behavioural changes among the affected individuals and communities. This is made possible because the stakeholders participate in the health communication design, development and implementation, which leads to better communication and to greater ownership of the communication goals and objectives. Today, health issues are a major agenda in the world and need to be addressed urgently by using innovative teaching methods.

Bibliography

Arntson, A.E. 1997. *Graphic Design Basics*. Oxford University, London.

Chandra, A., Shah, A. and Joshi, U. 1989. *Fundamentals of Teaching Home Science*. Sterling Publishers, New Delhi.

Chaudery, K.C. and Sachdev, J.L. 1996. *Total Literacy by 2000*. Indian Adult Education Association, New Delhi.

Kochar, S.K. 1990. *Methods and Techniques of Teaching*. Sterling Publishers, New Delhi.

Kumar, K. 1995. *Media Education Communication and Public Policy: An Indian Perspective*. Himalaya Publications, Delhi.

Ministry of Information and Broadcasting. 1993. Government of India Annual Report.

Nair, K.S. and White, S.A. 1993. *Perspectives on Development Communication*. Sage Publications, New Delhi.

Nicholas, C.B. and Carlos, A.T. 2006. *Globalization and Education: An Introduction*. Spencer Publications, London.

Roy, G.L. 1991. *Extension Communication and Management*. Naya Prakashan, Calcutta.

Singhal, A. and Verett, M.R. 1989. *Information Revolution*. Sage Publications, New Delhi.

Supe, S.V. 1991. *Introduction to Extension Education*. Oxford University Press, New Delhi.

6 Use of Folk Media in Health Education

It is very important to understand the diverse teaching materials, methods and media that have been developed to suit the requirements of different environments. Unfortunately, the field of literacy education has chronically lacked sound, comprehensive and comparative data – particularly on impacts – on which to establish conclusions and inferences for good organizational strategies and teaching methods. Education is closely associated with purposeful and organized social intervention programmes in the broader spectrum of human resource development. India has one of the largest educational networks in the world, but ironically, it also has the highest number of illiterates. Education sharpens the eye of knowledge, develops awareness and makes the mind logical. Without proper education, the scope and extent of the process of socio-economic changes cannot be understood by common men and they cannot take part in the process of development. Folk media is the best answer to this need for development. An inbuilt characteristic of folk media is that it is community based, uses the language and natural art of the community, and is not very expensive. At the same time, it is very powerful in convincing people and thus can act as a tool for conveying developmental messages to people living in rural and urban slums.

Definitions

Folk means people in general or as a mass. Folk includes a culture which already exists or is present and which is not new. It denotes the culture or traditions of a community of people, including their attitudes, beliefs, values, skills and thinking.

Any process, when used to disseminate knowledge, information and entertainment for a specific purpose, becomes media.

Combining the above two definitions, we can say that when we use cultural folk traditions and practices to provide knowledge and information to people, we get folk media. Folk media is sometimes identified with the rural or peasant people of a country. Folk media exists in all classes of society. Sometimes, the folk in question are a particular ethnic group or nationality. Folk media is part of folk culture. And the culture's lore, including its ballads and stories, is passed down by word of mouth from generation to generation. Different folk cultures, sometimes referred to as folk communities, developed in isolated areas where there was limited outside contact. The people within these communities worked to preserve their traditional cultural values.

Advantages of Folk Media over Electronic Media

Folk media is the media of the people because it has been with them for centuries and is a part of their lives. Folk media always has its own language, so it represents the community's true culture. As a result, the members of the community associate easily with its gestures, music and rhythm and understand it well. This characteristic of folk media develops familiarity, which is not possible with electronic media such as radio and television, where the sender and the receiver are unable to develop a personal rapport.

Folk media is less expensive and governments can use this art form to convey developmental messages to extend health education. Folk media has an added advantage over electronic media as the cost of developing it into an effective communication tool is extremely cost effective. It does not require electricity transmitters, receivers or technical experts.

Moreover, folk media employs the background, myths and legends which stem from the community's own region. Since folk media enjoys a high appeal, it leads to people participating actively in the communication process. As we know effective communication is the cornerstone for developing human relationships and exchanging thoughts and knowledge. Communication leads to the movement of knowledge and, therefore, to an exchange of knowledge, skills and attitudes between people and social groups. The objective of developmental communication is to bring about desirable change in the behaviour of people, and in this, folk media enjoys a significant advantage over electronic media.

A fundamental principle of human communication is that transfer of ideas occurs most frequently between sources and receivers who are alike or similar. This principle also makes folk media a most appropriate media because it enables immediate and constant feedback and the communicators can use the reactions of the receivers as a check for the effectiveness of current or future action. Folk media enjoys high credibility because the community perceives it to be trustworthy. Thus, it can be used very effectively for conveying developmental messages and people can be persuaded to act as change agents for the adoption of innovations. While planning programmes for rural development, it is important to blend media, with an emphasis on folk media, keeping the originality of each folk form and making it an integral part of the whole programme. Rural audiences understand folk media and are attracted to it; so, if health messages are incorporated through such media, it will be very effective, provided the collaboration between the folk artists and media producers is strong.

Role of Universities in Promotion of Health through Folk Media

Universities can do a lot of work for the promotion of good health in India. The process of involving the university system to participate in extension programmes was initiated by the University Grants Commission (UGC) with the specific objective of securing equal importance to extension education as the third dimension, along with teaching and research.

The infrastructure of higher education provides a large reservoir of human energy and resources. It is, therefore, imperative to mobilize the resources for nation building activities and utilize the infrastructure for national development to achieve the desired objectives. The system of education, especially higher education, in India has not been shaped to enable certain sections of society to acquire technological, organizational, managerial, sociological and cultural development. It is important that we prepare the appropriate teaching-learning materials, utilize effective teaching-learning methods and identify the appropriate loci for the teaching-learning process.

Generally speaking, there are three models through which a university and community could come together for 'learning' and for solving problems.

Models

- *The intra-institutional approach:* This model would incorporate the community's problems and the sociology of critical groups as part of the restructured syllabi at the graduate and postgraduate levels, so that all those going through formal education will have a chance to know, feel and realize their community and its needs.
- *University going to the masses:* This model involves the students and faculty moving to the community periodically, to be part of a service delivery system.
- *Action research:* This model links the university to the problems of the community for the purpose of solving its problems. It is possible for a democratically sensitive university system to establish this vital link between the educational system and traditional artisans. With their pre-existing technological orientation and background, the artisans would be in a better position than many other deprived sections to absorb the benefits of superior technological, managerial, organizational and socio-cultural capabilities, if the educational system is made accessible to them in an effective and relevant manner. There is a need to improve the total quality of their lives in the changing and emerging new settings and challenges of society in order to

ensure their survival and development, and health is one of the most critical of these challenges.

Academicians

As academicians, teachers can play a vital role by guiding students to take up action projects related to folk media. They can take up studies and research and provide invaluable help by carrying out research studies. Social scientists can create awareness about the importance of good health among the community people for their better future and progress, and thereby that of the nation, thus improving educational levels all round. In India, due to the rigid social structure, girls are not given proper food and nutrition, they are married off at an early age and they start bearing children soon after – all these factors lead to their dropping out of the formal educational system. Early marriage and the ensuing child bearing pose health risks for both themselves and their babies. Social scientists can help to convince people about the importance of health education and the dynamics of gender and health education. Teachers can tell students about the various folk media. They can guide and train students and interest them in folk media, leading to them adopting the media later in a more professional form. Teachers must assure a wide role in development work of extending knowledge, creating the scientific temper in communities, and actively participating in various health programmes. Teachers can contribute through techno-pedagogic inputs by means of organizing workshops, providing technical support and preparing database information related to health and folk media.

Communicators

As communicators, home scientists can impart education in both rural areas and among urban slum communities. Home scientists can use *bhavai* and puppet shows to convey health messages. University teachers can write scripts and manuals for imparting health education through folk media and in developing, using and harnessing folk media in the field because folk media is a powerful instrument for creating a suitable climate in favour of sensitizing people about the need for good health. Teachers can prepare training manuals for folk media and help in the preparation of training packages for folk media. As communicators, teachers can help in mass motivation and mobilization by creating mass awareness, building the right environment, spreading messages through students, mobilizing voluntary agencies and sharing success stories related to health education.

Researchers

Research in the field of folk media has been a neglected area so far. However, scientists can play an active role by carrying out research studies in thrust areas such as surveys to find out the different types of folk media and their experts in a region and to document the experts and their areas of expertise. Experimental studies to check on the effectiveness of different folk media are another possible research area. As home scientists work as extension workers too, they can become a link between the folk media experts in a community and health agencies. Research and analysis can be undertaken to assess the ways in which folk media reach and affect people. The outreach of different folk media by age, sex and occupation can be assessed. The reasons for the low use of folk media can be identified by universities. Evaluation studies can be undertaken by universities for qualitative improvement of folk media and its use for developmental purposes.

Non-formal Educators

The great challenge for humanity is to live with nature and technological changes. That is why universities and other academic institutions must create proper linkages between information technology and people. The Department of Home Science, Extension and Communication in a university can undertake different activities such as organizing seminars, symposia and debates on folk media and organizing field trips for students to enable them to study different folk media. A comprehensive training programme can be developed so that students acquire the skills and knowledge essential in the use of folk media. Training programmes can be organized to meet folk artists and master craftsmen and seek their cooperation in understanding folk media. Fairs, *shivirs*, health camps and *jathas* can be organized and folk media used in them to reach out to disadvantaged groups and impart health education.

Suggestions

- Both master craftsmen and teachers who are used to conventional media and methods should be encouraged and used as change agents.
- NGOs should be supported adequately to share the responsibility for the preservation, dissemination and documentation of cultural heritage and folk media for the promotion of health.
- A network of institutions is necessary to set high standards for training, support and strengthening of folk media and health education.
- PRIs and NGOs must be employed in the development and utilization of folk media for health messages.
- Folk art groups, comprising students, functionaries and local youth, should be set up with the help of talented folk artists to impart health education.
- Institutes should be equipped with adequate human resources such as qualified and competent health educators who have both theoretical insight and practical knowledge of folk media. This will enable correct training for students who, in turn, will act as change agents.
- Suitable steps should be taken by folk media practitioners to utilize the services of other forms of media to reach their target groups. Folk songs and stories should be printed as booklets and circulated widely.
- CDs should be made on the basis of scripts prepared through workshops. These scripts should be documented for wider publicity and used by different agencies and individuals for motivation and training.

- NGOs should be asked to help and encouraged to work in the field of health education.
- Volunteers should be enlisted and enrolled to act as 'master trainers'.
- Alternative media forms, such as folk theatre and puppet shows, should be encouraged widely, especially where the existing electronic and print media have no or limited outreach, such as in rural areas.
- After exposure to the folk media, the reactions of the target group should be extensively researched and analysed.
- Resource centres should be set up at the Central and state levels for identification, collection, dissemination and documentation of material related to folk media.

Conclusion

Audio-visual aids, which are relatively inexpensive, easily available, easy to prepare, carry, use and store, and which bring about the greatest clarity in learning, should be given priority in imparting health education. One has to be realistic about which objectives are immediately achievable and which will take more time to achieve. The current situation, which arises out of a reduced use of traditional low cost media and unavailability of modern electronic technology, must be worked around in order to achieve genuine growth. In India, which is still a developing country, a mixture of traditional and sophisticated media can serve the purpose. Folk media has its own strengths and characteristics and it has certain domains where it is stronger than any other media. Folk media helps to improve the process of human learning, which is a complex integrated process involving people, procedures and ideas, and devising, evaluating and managing solutions to the health problems faced by communities in the country. Imparting health education to disadvantaged groups is not an easy task because the people in such groups lack confidence in their ability to learn. But folk media, which is familiar to them, can be used to introduce both education and the importance of education to disadvantaged groups. In sheer monetary terms, the electronic mass media are of limited relevance to the masses, especially those who are living below the poverty line, who can barely meet their essential needs of food, clothing and shelter. Buying a cheap transistor set is a luxury they cannot afford and newspapers and periodicals are out of the question. Thus, widespread access to media and to media exposure cannot be expected among rural people, slum dwellers and other deprived sections of society. In such circumstances, folk media have far reaching consequences and can be an effective vehicle of social change. Universities and colleges have to take active part in this task of eradicating disease. As their effective participation is the need of the hour, no time should be lost in making traditional folk media a tool for developmental communication. Thus, folk media can help in the fight against illiteracy and in the promotion of good health.

Bibliography

Agarwal, J.C. 2000. *Principles, Methods and Techniques of Teaching.* Vikas Publishing House, New Delhi.

Dahama, O.P. and Bhatnagar, O.P. 1994. *Education and Communication for Development.* Oxford and IBH Publishing, New Delhi.

Goran, Hedebro. 1982. *Communication and Social Change in Developing Nations: A Critical View.* Iowa State University Press.

Kumar, Keval J. 1994. *Mass Communication in India.* Jaico Publishing House, Mumbai.

Mathur, K.B. 1990. *Communication for Development and Social Change.* Allied Publishers, Lucknow.

Nimbalkar, M.R. 1987. *Adult Education and Its Evaluation Systems.* Mittal Publications, Delhi.

Pillai, P. Ramachandra. 2004. *Non-Formal Education.* Neelkamal Publications Pvt. Ltd., New Delhi.

Prabha, Inder. 1988. *Adult Education in India: A Policy Perspective.* N.B.O. Publishers Distributors, Chandigarh.

Rafi, Kothar. 1984. 'Communication for Alternative Development', in *Development Dialogue*, Vol. 1–2.

Ramabrahman, I. 2005. *Adult Education Policy and Performance.* Gyan Publishing House, New Delhi.

Reddy, Vikram P. 1994. 'A Vanishing Art', in *The Hindu*, 27 February.

Shah, Anupama and Joshi, Uma. 1992. *Puppetry and Folk Drama for Non-Formal Education*. Sterling Publishers, New Delhi.

Yadav, Rajendra Singh. 2000. *Adult Education, Training and Productivity*. The Indian Publications, Ambala Cantt.

7 Field Trips for Non-Formal Education

Field trips, if handled skilfully, are an effective teaching technique. Field trips are excursions or visits for educational purposes to locations other than the regular classroom – an educational activity in which students leave the classroom and go out into the community to the actual source of information, that is, in logical extension of bringing part of the world into the classroom, the class is taken into the 'real' world. By gathering information firsthand, by actually seeing and experiencing, learning is more pleasurable and more accurate, interest is increased and there is a satisfying common experience. Field trips are useful not only because they give students firsthand knowledge and enable them to see how a number of skills and processes blend into a whole, but also because they can be used to provide students with cultural experiences available in no other way. Many students, for example, would never get to see the printing of a newspaper from start to finish unless they saw it on a field trip. Similarly, many students might never to go to an art museum or a basket making class unless they are introduced to them on a field trip. In short, we can say that field trips are a planned visit to points outside the classroom or the meeting place of the organization. They may also be defined as excursions organized by teachers to enrich the learning experience.

Confirmatory field trips serve as reinforcement for previously occurred learning, while exploratory field trips fulfil the basic function of discovery. Each approach is a structured attempt to provide an on the spot observation of some specific process, undertaking or activity.

Plans for field trips must be thorough and definite in order to avoid confusion and wastage of time. Generally, a field trip should be correlated with the unit of study and a thorough background should be prepared for the event before it takes place. It is helpful to prepare with the help of the class a list of relevant questions or items in order to fix and unify the experiences which the learners have had. If possible, the discussions may be conducted during the field trip or immediately after it.

Definition

Field trips are journeys by a group of people to places away from their normal environment. The purpose of such trips is usually observation, a non-experimental form of quantitative research. The aim of this research is to observe the subject in its natural state and possibly collect samples. In Western cultures, people first came across this method during school years, when classes were taken on excursions to visit, for example, a geological or geographical feature of the landscape. Much of the early research into the natural sciences was of this form. Charles Darwin is an important example of someone who has contributed to the sciences through the use of field trips in schools. Field trips are educational trips made by a class that normally last a day, but can be longer. Field trips usually consist of visits to local landmarks and educational places, such as zoos, parks and museums, including health museums.

All the rich resources of the community become available to children when they go together on excursions or field trips away from the classroom and into the immediate neighbourhood, nearby communities or distant parts of the country. Field trips seek to provide emotional meaning to otherwise purely verbal knowledge and to lead children into an understanding of the distinctive values of a community.

The National Centre for Research and Vocational Education defines field trips as visits to places outside the regular classroom designed to achieve certain objectives that cannot be achieved as well as by using other means.

Purpose and Value of Field Trips

- They provide firsthand and direct experience of the existing situation to students through observation.
- They motivate students to learn as they have opportunities to examine new materials and acquire new ideas.
- They acquaint students with their environment.
- They give students actual practice in purposeful planning and execution.
- They capitalize educationally the migratory instinct of man.
- They help to interpret, supplement and enrich curricular experiences.
- They give students actual practice in purposeful planning and execution.

Types of Field Trips

There are four types of field trips:

Local School Trips

These are the simplest kind of field trips. The group visits several points, parts and sections of their own school building and ground. This trip can be used for measuring distances, lying on the ground to play, plotting for demonstration, practising health and safety procedures, studying nature, watching, studying, and checking traffic posts and practising safety on the streets. These field trips are arranged during regular school periods. They do not cost money.

Community Trips

These field trips are conducted to show farms, fishery ponds, libraries, museums, a railway station or other destinations outside the school. They usually take half a day or a day or two at the most. These trips are often taken during the regular school week.

Tours

These are journeys or trips lasting several days, a month or even an entire season. Such trips are usually made to a distant place. They are undertaken by small groups for judging teams, prize winners, exhibitors and contestants as well as by large groups for studying an ongoing process or a large organization. The responsibilities for this type of trip are greater, the expenses heavier and the planning, organizing and execution more complicated.

Imaginary Tours

In such field trips, a single pupil takes a trip by himself due to some assigned responsibility or as a co-curricular activity. Such trips are brought about by one's own specialized interest. Through these trips, the pupil learns to recognize, appreciate, accept and discharge responsibilities complementary to education.

Choosing a Site

There are a number of things to consider when selecting a site that best suits the needs and requirements of a particular field trip. These considerations may include:

The suitability of different sites with respect to curriculum needs and its outcomes: For example, the presence of different types of ecosystems and/or the level of biodiversity in an area (for an ecological study) or the presence of examples of different types of land use (for resource management issues).

The time of year chosen for field trips poses a number of different problems, including likelihood of rain and the temperature extremes that can be expected – this will determine the appropriateness of clothing and other equipment as well as the enjoyment of the trip.

The existence of local experts at the site, such as park rangers and/or the presence of visitors' centres and displays, may provide additional learning experiences. The organizers must decide whether to utilize the resources of the education centres and visitors' centres in addition to their own staff and equipment. The presence or otherwise of facilities such as bus parking, toilets and lunch areas is also important.

Procedural Steps

Identification of the Units of Study

Ensure that the topic selected is appropriate for field trip observations. The excursion should be the best approach for the learning experience and it should satisfy the unit's established objectives.

Planning

Good preliminary planning is the most vital factor for successful field trips. The students can be asked to help in determining the place of visit. Select several possible locations to be visited. Make the necessary arrangements with the people involved. Check all the details of the facilities, time and other considerations. Work out what is to be observed with the sponsoring organization. Develop a definite time schedule including departure, observation and return. Visit the establishment beforehand, if possible.

Administrative and Organizational Details

Obtain the permissions of the administration for the field trip. Distribute and get back parental permission slips from each participating student. Provide for suitable transportation if required. Make provisions for food, whenever necessary.

Preparation

Generally outline and discuss what to look for during the field trip. Indicate any special clothing to be worn or materials to be worn or materials to be included on the excursion. Caution the class about any safety precautions or general rules and regulations which should be followed. As a group, identify some possible questions that might arise.

Conducting the Field Trip

Ensure that there is adequate supervision. Keep a close watch on the movements of the group to avoid straying or misconduct. Be prepared to answer questions as they arise or to enlist the assistance of the person in charge of the visit. Provide for a certain amount of freedom for the students.

Discussion

Arrange for letters of appreciation to be sent to the sponsoring individuals or organization. Enlist student participation in this courtesy. Facilitate a meaningful discussion of the experience. Outline the main ideas and summarize the observations. Develop other student activities as an outgrowth of the excursion. Allow students to assist in an appraisal of the field trip.

Planning

- Determine the students' accessibility to the site – distance and availability of transportation (walking, cars or buses).
- Assess the area for any safety considerations, such as loose rocks, cacti, broken glass, etc.
- Check to determine if the site is appropriate for the activities planned.
- Determine the location of the nearest restroom, shelter and telephone.
- Secure approval from the owners of the site and from the school authorities.
- Speak with the host or guide, if applicable, and review the purpose of the trip and the activities planned.

Teachers' Preparation

- Send letters to parents/guardians explaining the purpose of the field trip, appropriate dress and requesting volunteers.
- Send permission slips to parents requesting medical information, name and phone number of health practitioners, phone numbers for emergencies and the parents' and students' signatures.
- Contact parent volunteers and explain their responsibilities during the day's activities.
- Plan post-trip activities to follow up on the field trip activities.

- Gather material needed for the trip, such as magnifying glasses, clipboards, extra pencils, crayons, thermometers, etc.
- Gather material for a group leader backpack, which should include:
    - First aid kit
    - Extra water bottle
    - Extra hat
    - Extra paper and pencils
    - Sunscreen
    - Mobile phone
    - Extra snacks
    - Permissions slips for students

Preparing the Students for a Field Trip

- Discuss the purpose of the field trip and how it relates to the current unit of study.
- Introduce visual observation skills, Let students describe in detail ordinary objects, such as a paper clip, paintbrush, clothes peg or comb, to their classmates.
- Show photographs or posters of the field trip site or related to the exhibits that will be viewed.
- Assign various students 'specialist' roles in one aspect of the topic that they will be studying during the field trip. Students could be grouped to research the different subject areas related to the field trip.
- Explore the website of the location you will be visiting.
- Organize a class brainstorming session to come up with a set of conduct standards for the trip and discuss spending money, lunch plans, appropriate clothing to wear for the trip, including rain gear.
- Discuss with the students how to ask good questions and brainstorm on a list of open ended observations and questions to help gather information during the visit. Record questions on chart paper or in student field trip journals.
- Overview the field trip schedule.

Students' Preparation

Introduce the students to the purpose of the trip and the activities in which they will be engaged during the trip.

- Plan activities that introduce content, such as the pre-trip activities set out in Ecosystem Explorations.
- Establish expectations of appropriate behaviour by doing an activity such as the Goal Setting lesson in Ecosystem Explorations.
- Demonstrate the appropriate methods of use for all the equipment that will be used.
- Divide the class into teams and give each team or child specific tasks to be responsible for during the field trip.

During Field Trips

- Remember that teachers and adult volunteers serve as guides throughout the day to facilitate learning by the students.
- Divide the class into smaller groups and assign each group to an adult volunteer.
- Plan for restroom breaks immediately prior to departure and throughout the day.
- Do a head count at each stop and make sure that an adult is at the front and end of the line while hiking.
- Keep the activities varied and allow for sufficient time for observation and reflection.
- Focus on keeping the activities student centred by encouraging student inputs and participation.
- Reflect on the pre-trip objectives during the trip to determine when to remain flexible and adapt your activities to fit the needs of your group, the weather and the time available.

Do's and Don'ts for Field Trips

- Do not plan impulsive, spur of the moment trips.
- Do survey all trip possibilities in your local area.
- Do plan each detail of the trip carefully.
- Do use the trip for job training.
- Do make certain that the students know what to observe.

- Do prepare guide sheets for each trip.
- Do prepare the students for the trip.
- Do observe punctuality.
- Do work in small groups.
- Do correlate the trip with specific training jobs.
- Do prepare photographs, slides or motion pictures of the trip.
- Do follow up on the trip as soon as possible.
- Do use pictures, slides and motion pictures for review purposes.
- Do test the students.
- Do evaluate and check the results of each trip.
- Do catalogue and file all trip material for future reference.

Follow-up

Proper follow-up is very necessary and important step in making field trips successful. This involves writing thank you letters to the host and everyone who helped in making the trip a success, apart from the students. Also:

- Brainstorm with the students: What did we learn? What did we do? Have them share that information with their families or another class.
- List ideas or questions that were raised or left unanswered during the trip.
- Expand on the field trip by relating the experience to classroom activities by using Ecosystem Explorations or other activities.
- File a short report on the field trip to use for future reference, including factual information about the site used and contacts as well as evaluation of the activities.

Evaluating Field Trips

Field trips can be evaluated by conducting discussions using the following pointers:

- Did the field trip serve the purpose for which it was intended?

- What are the factors that accounted for its success?
- Was there sufficient time to observe what was planned?
- Were the routes and means of transportation satisfactory?
- What changes are necessary if the same place is to be visited again?

Advantages

- Field trips can provide information that is not to be obtained in books. They can add a dimension of reality and interest that makes the school curriculum a living thing because field trips help in getting firsthand information.
- When it becomes important to teach community values leading to improved behaviour in students, then economy of time cannot be considered the most important factor.
- Almost any field trip holds the probability of content, people and pleasant experiences in kind behaviour.
- Students also get acquainted with another school, people of another race and aged people, who cannot come to their school, but have a vivid memory of folklore and community history.
- Free expression and a field trip will often result in creative writing, individual paintings and group murals, musical compositions and other forms of expression.
- Field trips can influence students' emotions.
- They may help students in selecting their life work.
- Field trips to rural areas can help students to understand rural life.
- They can provide opportunities for gaining new experiences and information.
- They enable the observation of objects in their natural setting.
- They enable the observation and stimulation of students' interest and keenness.
- They provide opportunities for learning by doing.
- They enable the observation and stimulation of concrete and realistic events, which cannot be had in the classroom.

- They help in developing unity of purpose among the students.
- They serve as an excellent stimulant for participating in later discussions or activities.
- They help to bridge the gap between the school and the community and the gulf that often exists between different subjects in the curriculum. They also afford opportunities for exploration, investigation and discovery in real life situations, which amplify and extend theoretical study.

Disadvantages

Field trips require a lot of planning by the teacher and coordination with the students and the hosts of the place where the trips will be undertaken.

- If the teacher is unable to create understanding of why the trip is being undertaken and what to look for on the trip, then a field trip has no meaning.
- School field trips are usually tied in with the requirement of the curriculum, but, at times, do not fulfil the stated aims.
- Field trips may become extremely time consuming and costly and must be continually evaluated in the light of educational values.

Conclusion

Field trips are a beautiful part of educational activity. In addition to all the advantages discussed earlier, they also improve school-community relations by increasing interaction between the two. Field trips and the use of outside speakers both provide interaction and thus help to improve school-community relations.

Bibliography

Atkinson, F.W. and Rogner, F. 1972. *Achievement Motivation.* V.M. Winston & Sons, Washington DC.

Bhargava, M. and Sakia, L.R. 2005. *Teachers in the 21st Century.* Rakhi Prakashan, Agra.

Bruce, Joyce and Well, Marsha. 1985. *Models of Teaching*. Prentice Hall of India, New Delhi.

Erickson, E.H. 1979. *Childhood and Society*. W.W. Norton & Co., New York.

Howard, E.H. 1979. *Teaching in Middle Schools*. International Textbook Co., Pennsylvania.

Levin, K. 1988. *The Social Context*. Oxford University Press, London.

Line, H. and Beauchamp, M. 1959. *Human Relations in Teaching*. Prentice Hall Inc., New York.

Modi, B. 1991. *Designing Messages for Development*. Sage Publications, New Delhi.

Paralikar, K. 1990. *The Art of Teaching Home Science*. Ekvira Publication, Vadodara.

Roy, Aruna (Ed.) 1984. *Education of Out-of-School Children: Case of Selected Non-formal Learning Programmes of South Asia*. Commonwealth Secretariat, London.

Sandhu, A.S. 1996. *Textbook of Agricultural Communication: Process and Methods*. IBH Publishing, New Delhi.

Singh, L.C. 1995. *Multiple Models of Teaching for Educators*. Vikas Publishing House, New Delhi.

Suzanne, K. 1990. *Non-Formal Education: An Empowering Process*. Center for International Education, 285 Hills, USA.

Water, Pierce D. and Lorber, Michael A. 1979. *Objectives and Methods for Secondary Teaching*. Prentice Hall International Inc., London.

8 Games for Differently Abled Children

Education aims to bring about desirable changes in people in order to promote their adjustment with their environment. The fundamental aim of education is the physical, intellectual, emotional and ethical evolution of an individual into a complete man. In another light, it can be said that you can see both a collective and an individual aspect in the aim of education. Modern psychological research has recognized this complex task of education. Education develops the creative faculties only when, as Froebel put it, children are treated as flowers growing in a garden and encouraged to develop inquisitive and open minds. As Rabindranath Tagore said, "Growth is the movement of a whole towards a fuller wholeness". Living things possess this wholeness from the beginning. A child has its own perfection as a child. Since, in the formal learning situation, the end product is predefined, planning for as well as coordinating and controlling of experience to reach the ends is easier. However, in extension education, which is need based and 'flexible' in nature, it becomes difficult to plan and execute learning experiences in a 'tailor-made' fashion.

The most commonly dealt with beneficiary group under home science extension activities are children, youth, especially young girls, and adult women. Very little work has been done on the needs and learning of children with special needs in the community and how to impart non-formal education to them. Most programmes for young children with special needs make provision for the continuing education of those who provide education to them and who are closely related to them in their daily routine life. It is important to know how to choose and the types of games that might be useful for extension educators working with student trainees and teachers of children with special needs or even with the parents and siblings of such children or an organization for such children in the community.

With the growing sense of 'groups' in the social development of primary children, games play an important role in the physical education programme. But with our growing understanding of the value of free play in an arranged environment, games are also good for developing sturdy, skilful bodies; movement explorations and rhythms are valuable in helping children discover the range of flexibility of their own body movements. In the light of all these insights, games are more important in the total education programme than ever before. On the other hand, with our growing understanding of the importance of daily physical education, children's total experience with games will not be reduced materially; in many cases, other activities will be extended greatly.

Games may be classified as running and chasing games, circle games, ball games and singing games. Each has its own particular value for children. Lack of resources and timetable constraints may make it difficult for teachers to introduce gaming simulation in its full form. They may also feel that their students are not ready to cope with the organizational, linguistic and social demands of the method.

Card, board and group games are widely used with vocational preparation, partly on the grounds that an activity that is 'fun' will be accepted more easily than a formal lesson. Games can help to foster group cohesion. And games and games-like activities, into which the language items to be practised are woven, can weave in the extended context by various other means Then, as soon as learners can read something in the foreign language for themselves, the extended context is provided by the whole printed piece, as, for example, by a whole story. In the early stages of a foreign language course, it is the pictured story that is needed, and in that we have one of the chief uses of pictures in foreign language teaching.

The games that are thought of when people mention 'play in learning' are loosely organized activities that have elements of competition, individual skill, chance and drill. Games are a natural way for children to express their feelings. The play therapy situation is one in which children are given an opportunity to 'play out' their problems, much as an adult may 'talk out' his difficulties with friends, a doctor or a therapist.

A game is an educational play situation that possesses some structure by virtue of a set of rules or procedures that have to be followed. Games may require varying degrees of skill, concentration and coordination, depending upon their organization and execution.

According to Dr Wriston, "A game is an activity in which participants follow prescribed rules that differ from those of reality as they strive to attain a challenging goal."

According to Jay B. Nash, "A game is the administrative or teaching division of education that is concerned with vigorous total body activities as distinct from manual, musical and science activities." The aims of the games are personal development, increased confidence and assertiveness, and empathy with others. Used carefully, they can promote cooperation, tone down dominating students and draw out the quieter ones. They can lead to heightened self-knowledge and personal growth in general. However, the play has to be finished before the discussion can start, so timing is important. "What do I want my students to learn from playing this?" is of prime and utmost importance.

The word, 'game', comes from an old Teutonic word meaning 'joy'. It denotes an activity that is indulged in for the sake of the pleasure it offers, rather than any set purpose. It achieves in a narrower sense of contest carried out according to the rules and decided by the strength, skill or luck of the contestants, as who will win the game or who will loose. Games are educational play situations possessing some structure by virtue of sets of rules to be followed. Games may require varying degrees of skill, concentration and coordination, depending upon their organization and execution. Games are a natural and essential element of human development. They are an important method by which knowledge, experience and entertainment can be provided in one go. Interest in games is a complex of instinctive tendencies that are a striking feature of human nature, not only of children, but also of adults, and one that cuts across social divisions. The interest of the affluent and better educated classes is illustrated by the fact that many of the leading daily newspapers, which focus on these classes, publish strong sports pages. The interest of children in games is proverbial as in the case of imitative play. Games of all kinds, minor expeditions and trips of exploration keep them absorbed and help to expend their energy.

Games should provide enough content experience for each player to justify the time spent playing them and should hold the active attention of all the players. Games offer learning through activities that have elements of competition, individual skills, change and physical experience. Thus, games are very useful in the extension teaching-learning process. But keep in mind that games should be changed as soon as interest slackens in the activity.

Choosing Games

Teachers must bear the following points in mind while evaluating games and simulations:

- Will the time required to use them fit into your schedule and your available time?
- Is the game you are considering a board or non-board game and will it be reusable?
- Will it fit the size of the class in which you would want to use it? If not, is it flexible enough to be adapted without losing its value as a learning resource?
- Is it too elaborate or too expensive for the purposes you seek to achieve?
- Is it a game to be used by individuals or small groups in a learning centre or is it better suited for large group learning situations?
- Are the directions for the game appropriate for your students or are they too complicated and time consuming?
- After deciding to use a simulation or a game, a helpful practice is to have a few students examine and play it before trying it out on the entire class.

Criteria for Selecting an Appropriate Game

- It should be a teaching device.

- It should have purpose with a specific type of development.
- It should provide enough content and experience for the players for the amount of time spent.
- It should hold the active attention of the players.
- It should be self-motivating and within the experience of the children.
- It should include a definite goal to be reached by an individual or a group.
- It should encourage a spirit of helpfulness and fair play among the participants.
- Sometimes, the basis of games should be charm rather than ability, so that opportunities are offered to children of varying ability to play together.

Characteristics of Games

Rules must be followed:

- Competition is created between individuals. The learner must take chances and take the consequences of each decision at the end of the game.
- A winner emerges at the end of the game.
- Games, particularly those that involve teamwork, encourage an emotionally disciplined state.
- Games should create a self-oriented approach in the learner.
- They are teaching-learning techniques in which students learn or practise what they have already learnt.
- Games offer a variety of play with entertainment purposes.
- Games provide physical and mental development to the learners.
- Games provide practical in-depth knowledge and experience to the learners.
- Games should be allotted to people of all ages.

Importance of Games

Perhaps more indicative of the importance of games is their role as a basis of learning many new and needed skills and insights. They are not simply recreational activities that provide exercise or fill time.

Rather, they enable students to learn to achieve specific goals or objectives in active mode

- Games increase the intelligence quotient of children and help in their mental development.
- They can be used for self-learning.
- They enable children to experience joy.
- They help to develop habits of fair play and good sportsmanship.
- They help to develop motor skills, good posture and good health.
- They help to quicken sensory perceptions.
- They help to establish both self-confidence and self-control.
- They help to get participants to cooperate as an integral part of a group.
- Most people enjoy setting aside the logical rules of everyday life and entering an artificial environmental with different dynamics.
- Both children and adults like to play.
- Children are usually happy to participate in recreational activities.
- Games should act as a reaching device and each game should target a specific type of development.
- The educational value of games lies in cultivating a spirit of true and chivalrous sportsmanship.
- A games format can be used to motivate both children and adults to practise and hone their intellectual skills.
- The learners should be physically, mentally and actively involved in the games.

Types of Games

Sensory Games

The early years of childhood offer us the most favourable opportunity for training and strengthening the senses and it is vital that this work should not be neglected. The wider the range of impressions, the richer will be children's early sensory experiences and the more favourable the conditions for their complete development. Games aid children in learning the names and characteristics of materials.

Social Games

Social games are very effective in teaching unselfishness, kindness, politeness and consideration for others. Children learn by doing, so they learn to be polite by actually speaking and behaving kindly and politely. Mere lectures and words will roll over children without having much influence on their conduct. Games reinforce the appeal made to their sympathies through their stories, translate feelings into deeds, and the repeated actions necessary in games leave indelible impressions on the mind.

Visiting Games

One family may visit another and, during the visit, the children are encouraged to talk to each other and to the teachers, who join in as freely and naturally as possible. Such games encourage conversation and tend to minimize shyness and awkwardness.

Nature Games

Nature games, which are defined as the life of the world around man, hold a strong fascination for young children. Hence, the prominence given to nature sequel of which should be increased interest in the world of nature and the development of more definite ideas with regard to the objects discussed e.g., it can be trees, leafs, animals or birds. Nature games should be the spontaneous expression of impressions gained during nature talks – the dramatic outcome, which is an especially fitting means of expressing themselves.

Group Games

Group games help to create group oriented feelings in children. It is important to make the aim of such games clear to all players, provide them with full knowledge of the game, and to keep scores because this will be a source of motivation.

Running and Chasing Games

Games that involve running and chasing are among the best for children of early primary school age. They contribute especially to the development of leg muscles, to the children's skill in dodging and to their speed in moving. Kin-mine is a skill in which the six-year-old has gained confidence. Elements that encourage speed are not avoided, nor are they emphasized. Games of this kind usually involve a large number of children in activity at the same time. This high involvement contributes to the development of a larger number of children than games that require long waits for each child's turn. On the other hand, such games generally need a device by which the individual child can check himself out inconspicuously and rest on a self-demand basis. A 'safe' area is desirable when the game involves continuous running or the threat of being chased.

Games of this kind fall into a number of categories with different names and slight variations, such as Brownies and Fairies, Run, Sheep, Run, and Squirrel in the Tree.

Circle Games

A circle formation in games is conducive to control and contributes an element of unity. Often, these elements of control and unity are important for the time in which the games are being played, as at the beginning of the school year, or when the group needs to be ready for the next activity on immediate call. On the other hand, circle games tend to have a limited number of children active at one time. This decreases body building value. Individual children may help maintain the circle formation that makes the game possible for the entire playing time, yet not have an opportunity for active participation.

Most six year olds, after a little practice, can be effectively cooperative in forming a circle. The group habit of forming a small circle first, standing close together so that no arms have to be stretched, makes the process easier. Circle games also fall into groups according to different patterns with slight variations in their rules. They include Drop the Handkerchief, Slap Jack, and Cat and Rat.

Team Games

Team games are games in which children are divided into teams. Such games teach children how to play as a team, how to follow rules and how to play in a disciplined manner. It is probably true that children who benefit from team games would play them whether they were compulsory or not, and that those who are forced to play them are unlikely to benefit from them. A better solution is to provide alternative forms of socialized physical activity for non-game-playing pupils, such as Scouting or Guiding, cycling, hiking, camping, field studies, school journeys and folk dancing.

Singing Games and Folk Dancing

Singing games are a quieter type of game – the maximum involvement of the children is in the music and usually in the actions that accompany it. As another form of rhythmic action, these game stand in close relation to folk dances, which the children will begin to start gradually. Although structured in action and limited in opportunities for skill development, they are an important factor in children's cultural heritage and their timeless spirit should be a part of all children's experiences. Children should not be urged to sing more loudly for the game, but all of them should be encouraged to sing. If the action of the singing game is fast or strenuous, it is desirable to have music on or allow the children to take turns in both acting and singing. Some examples of singing games are little red worm painted blue, Looby Loo, and Round and Round the Village.

Ball Games

A variety of ball games are suitable for children. Such games may require activities such as throwing, kicking, bouncing and passing. Children learn quickly that ball games are more fun when all the players cooperate.

Games can be classified as

- Those involving bodily activity.
- Those involving little or no bodily activity.

Game Involving Bodily Activity

Such games involve a good amount of physical activity on the part of the player. They help in reducing the inner pent-up energy of children and keep them relaxed. These games are divided into the following categories:

- *Imitative games:* In these games, the children imitate the leader. This increases their observation powers and keeps their minds active. For example, Looby Loo.
- *Choosing games:* In these games, each child chooses a person in the group with whom he/she will play the game. For example, a skipping game.
- *Dramatic games:* These games involve the dramatization of stories with which the children are familiar. For example, The Little Princess, and Five Little Chickadees.
- *Purely social games:* These games result in the social development of children because they involve all the participants and have to be played cooperatively. They do not involve any type of victory or defeat. All the participants get an equal chance at playing the game. For example, Postman, Beckoning Game, and Here We Go Walking.
- *Seeing or observing games:* These games involve the keen observation of children and proper memory recall. They involve colours, searching, recalling and observing. For example, Policeman and the Lost Child, and Finding a Friend.
- *Games of touch:* These games involve the perceptive abilities of children, who have to recognize items by touch, without seeing or hearing them. For example, identifying the various objects placed in a cloth bag, identifying a child counting, and putting beads into a bag.
- *Mental gymnastic games:* These games involves a kind of brainstorming or buzz session, in which children think through for themselves the next stage of the game and describe it in their own way to maintain the continuity of game. For example, Mrs Brown's Party, My Suitcase, and Do as I Say but Not as I Do.

- *Guessing games:* These games involve a high level of mental ability for they encourage children to guess the right answers by themselves from among a selection. For example, I am Too Small, and Who has the Button?
- *Games of motor skill:* These games involve jumping, running, skipping and stopping, and use acute motor skills. For example, Dodge Ball, Crossing the Stream, and Ring Toss.
- *Gymnastic or stunt games:* These games involve physical exercise and result in the proper physical development of the playing children. For example, bicycling, turning cartwheels, and getting up from the floor without using your hands.
- *Competitive games:* These are games in which one is the winner and the other is the loser. Such games help to develop a feeling of competitiveness among the players. For example, Drop the Handkerchief. Musical Chairs, and Touch Ball.

Games Involving Little or No Bodily Activity

These games are of a quieter sort, but there are not as many of them as the more active games. Such games quicken sensory perceptions and develop mental ability. They can be divided thus:

Hearing games: These games involve the grasping power of children because they involve playing by hearing. For example, Ring Bell Ring, Dog and the Bone, and Hunting for the Ball.

Value of Games

Although teachers have used games for centuries, the many new forms of simulation and game materials are often not familiar to them, and new bases for choosing them are still developing. However, there are some limited indications of their particular values.

The conditions under which simulation games are conducted are important. Students are more positive about games when they understand the instructor's purpose in using them. Simulation games can teach facts, concepts and relationships as effectively as conventional instruction with the same objectives.

In certain fields, such as vocabulary building and mathematics, both simulation and non-simulation games produce greater learning than conventional instruction. Generally, games increase student motivation. There are also indications that in both games and simulation activities, competition encourages students to help each other, especially students with different abilities or students of a different gender. The most conspicuous contribution of games appears to be in providing motivational support for learning and contributing, in some cases, to attitudinal changes.

Because of the wide variety of games, simulations and learning environments available, teachers and students must try out new games and simulations carefully in order to select those of the greatest value.

Advantages

- Games involve active participation on the part of the learners, so they learn by discovering new things.
- Games can be used for learning new technologies, modifying undesirable work abilities and applying learning imaginatively to new ideas.
- Competitive games provide an unusually satisfactory social outlet for the instinctive aggressive drive. Psychiatrists postulate the existence in the human personality of an aggressive instinct, which constantly seeks expression.
- Relaxation through entertainment also satisfies important psychological needs by catering to passive desires.
- Slow learners can be motivated to learn something new with the help of educational games.
- Games provide increased mental ability and creativity to the learners.
- Games are a means by which knowledge, experience and entertainment all meet together.
- Games are an important tool by which learners become self-reliant and group oriented.

Disadvantages

- Learners do not take games seriously as an educational tool; they often play games for merely entertainment purposes.
- All games are not universally suitable.
- Games are both expensive and time consuming.
- In the planning stage, the cooperative managerial and leadership skills and qualities are all tested and discussed as variations of the game, which leads to the game becoming tiring.
- Games should be changed from time to time, so that they do not become boring.
- They require a lot of time and skill.
- Complicated games are difficult for children to play.
- Some games require the constant presence of parents or teachers for correcting the children.

When to Use Games

- As ice breakers with new groups.
- As a way of getting an unsettled group to work together.
- When you want students to interact without using you as a medium.
- When you want to do something enjoyable with a group, particularly when you feel you do not get on well with them.
- When you want students to discover some ideas or information for themselves.

When Not to Use Games

As time fillers because this devalues the potential they offer as learning experiences.

With groups that are so unsettled that some students may seize the opportunities presented for disruption or to manipulate or make scapegoats of other students.

Suggestions for Games

- Schedule a regular time for playing games and have all the necessary equipment available so that each player can select, use and return what he needs.

- Use student leaders to teach others to play the games. Station each helper in an assigned area and have all those who wish to learn a particular game from a particular student helper go to that area.
- Walk around and visit all the areas as a friendly supervisor to help each student who needs assistance.
- Provide a wide variety of active and passive games.
- Increase participation and interest through tournaments, giving recognition to the winners and using as many student committees and as much assistance as possible.

Points to be Kept in Mind by Instructors

When you plan to use games for instruction, keep the following points in mind:

- Assess the readiness to learn for playing a selected game. Start by deciding whether the game will advance the achievement of the learners' objectives. Anticipate the questions that may arise when the game is played. Determine how much and what information must be given at the beginning of the game, choose the players, how the room should be arranged, and how to introduce the game.
- Find ways to adapt the games to the capabilities of the trainees. Keep in mind that many of the best and most successful simulation and other games from commercial sources are not delivered with every detail planned.
- Determine in advance whether to use all or only part of a game. Many classroom games involve at least two players or call for play by two or more teams because of the great amount of activity involved.

Maintain discipline. Announce the rules and regulations of the game so that all the learners can respect and follow them.

Be mindful of the safety precautions required for the game materials, equipment, and other factors such as time duration.

Supervising and Marketing

The instructors must supervise the game. Supervising provides the criteria of checking the learners' abilities. Instructors must mark points for each learner's activity so that perfect results are obtained from the game.

Keeping scores is very important because scores motivate learners to do well and learn well.

Evaluation

After giving the scores, instructors must evaluate the learners so that they get an idea of the learners' abilities and so that they can help them improve further.

Involving Parents in Behaviour Management Programmes

When parents or families are involved, any programme of behaviour change initiated at school can be carried home for further practice and supplementary teaching. This strengthens the behavioural change in children and increases their rate of learning Parental involvement in the teaching or training of children with disabilities increases the personal worth and sense of participation as the parents begin to feel more responsible for the fulfilment of their child's needs and requirements. Parents and families understand their child better than anyone else. This knowledge can be utilized by the teachers.

Conclusion

Games create interest in the learners. The playing of games is an age old tradition, but the games played and the way in which they are played have varied from time to time. Games are universally acknowledged as the best source of all types of development. Children should be introduced to various types of games from a very early age. Games should be included as a basic necessity in their lives. "These are the best source of utilization of time, learning enhancing in the capabilities."

Both the psychologist and the educationist agree on the valuable role played by games in children's lives. Games serve a recreational and educational purpose. They are an important tool by which learners acquire practical, in-depth knowledge and experience.

In extension education, games are a very approachable method because informal education creates democratic situations for learners.

Games provide learning by doing. They are very helpful in educating people of all ages, particularly those with mental and physical handicaps. Differently abled children are known to have more behavioural problems than their more normal counterparts. These problems may result from poor problem solving skills, cognitive and communication deficits or wrong handling by people in their environment. These problems must be managed as early as possible before they reduce the acceptability of children with special needs.

Teachers should identify learners and their goals. The teachers' objective is to make learning easier and more attractive. They should play and identify the resources that are used in games. They should list and describe the materials and arrangements required for planning games. Teachers should identify the principal rules of play and determine how players will interact and establish how and when the game is won. Teachers should also develop post-game evaluation.

Bibliography

Allen, Brent. 1978. *Philosophical Foundation for the Curriculum*. George Allen & Unwin, London.

Brown, James W., Lewis, Richard B., Harcleroad R. and Fred F. 1983. *A V Instruction, Technology Media Methods.* Fong & Sons Printers Pvt. Ltd., New York, USA, 6th edition, 2002.

Butterworth, Christine and MacDonald, Monica. 1985. *Teaching Social Education and Communication: A Practical Handbook.* Hutchinson, London.

Desai, D.C. 1990. *Patterns of Primary Education.* Harper & Row Publishers, New York.

Huey, J. Frances. 1987. *Teaching Primary Children.* Holt, Rinehart & Winston Inc., San Francisco.

Leonard, E.M. 1978. *Foundations of Learning in Childhood Education.* Charles E. Merrill Books, Chicago, USA.

Mansukhani, G.S. and Dhillon, G.S. 1973. *Whither Secondary Education?* Oxford & IBH Publishing Co., New Delhi.

Nash, J.B. 1991. *The Administration of Physical Education.* A.S. Barnes & Co., New York.

Nutting, W.C. 1976. *Designing Classroom Spontaneity*. Prentice Hall Inc., New Jersey.

Parker, S.C. 2001. *General Methods of Teaching in Elementary Schools*. Ginn & Co., Chicago.

Paterson, A.M. 1995. *A Handbook of Physical Activities and Games*. University of London Press Ltd., London.

Schonell, F.J. 1988. *The Psychology Teaching of Reading*. Oliver & Boyd, London.

9 Recreation for Children

Leisure is discretionary time or the time when people are free to do as they choose. The amount of leisure available can be isolated by a process of elimination if one begins with the total mass of time available to man. Deduct from the total those necessary activities that must be devoted to sustaining health: work to maintain an acceptable standard of living and obligations to maintain a family, and religious and civil duties. What is left is leisure, or spare time. However, there are other interpretations of leisure and its role. One concept sees leisure not merely as a time block, but as a force, which is not only the germinating concept of art and culture, but also a pause during which participants gain glimpses of values and realities that they miss ordinarily in everyday life. Such a perspective supports the proposition that the quality of civilization depends upon such a transmission of values. The widespread distribution and use of leisure is a matter of great importance to a nation – both culturally and economically.

Another somewhat aristocratic viewpoint treats leisure as a necessary condition of civilized life. In this theory, the ends of altruistic mankind are advanced by the leisure used, these ends being of a higher qualitative value and ultimately improving the higher, cultural tone of society. In turn, another theory calls leisure the purpose of work, with the idea that leisure activity may or may not be socially useful; instead, leisure contains singular, lofty qualities that make its use a reward in themselves.

The Nature of Recreation

What men do during their leisure has changed during the course of years and events. Changes in values, meanings and thinking have evolved primarily because of the overall development of the nation. People had a different meaning and purpose in fishing, hunting, hiking and canoeing during the earlier days of struggle to fashion homes and cities out of wilderness, and these were primarily methods of transport, subsistence and communication. Today, many of these efforts and experiences are defined as recreation. Recreation has come to exist in many different forms and meanings to different people. To understand its nature is to become familiar with a few of its salient characteristics as an experience.

Firstly, recreation should be recognized as an essential part of life. It is inescapable that time for leisure pursuits must be part of people's daily lives and, therefore, found in parts of the makeup of a family, living group or community. Man inherits play as a biological urge from childhood. This urge grows and develops into higher forms of activity, which find fruition in associations with other men. A fundamental knowledge of human behaviour ascertains the prominence of recreation among the basic activities of life. Next, recreation must be related to the interests and needs of an individual and geared for his own personal development. From this point, individuals' voluntary participation is geared directly towards their own recreational attitudes and frames of reference.

Recreation experiences can benefit the human personality. Recreation has constructive connotations of physical, mental and social characteristics for the personality. Therefore, it is accepted that by developing recreation skills and interests related to their individual drives, people can develop their personality favourably and make a positive contribution to society.

Finally, recreation exists in a multitude of activity forms. Its patterns appear based on a variety of desires, interests and pursuits. Recreational activities include music, drama, crafts, art, hobbies and reading as well as sports and physical activities. Even pursuits of a more serious nature such as civic participation and service, hobbies and study fall into the category of leisure.

Importance of Recreation

Since earlier times, recreation, like work, love and worship, has been an important aspect of living. Festivals, dances, games and music have always been a part of life, although at times they have been looked upon with disapproval by certain groups. Recreation plays a major role in people's lives. When the unrelenting pressure for survival shrouds human existence, as it does today, there is very little time to indulge in leisure activities. Recreation is meant for unburdening one's weary mind and body by spending time in a manner which is not gainful materially. Recreational activities may be of myriad types – sports and games, hobbies, vacations, and so on. Some forms of recreation can be more esoteric as well. The importance of recreation can be listed thus:

- It is a must to improve cognitive skills.
- It is beneficial in improving physical skills.
- It is needed to improve emotional well-being.
- It is useful in decreasing behavioural problems.
- It is needed to improve the health of individuals.

Interplay of Education and Recreation

Education and recreation are separate terms. However, some people claim that if the definition of education is broad enough, it can include recreation, but this renders unclear the difference between recreation and education. A contemporary view as expressed by Hutchinson accepts recreation as an integral part of the total educational process – his viewpoint is based on the idea that the learning process consists of components parts which can be applied in many recreational situations since the learning situation does not ultimately depend upon a particular type of institution or agency or their settings. Hutchinson reveals that actual educational principles can be applied readily to many recreational situations. These elements encompass the relationship of the individual to motivation, understanding, achievement and transfer of learning to another situation. Because of its informal character, recreation is urged as a method to achieve certain educational goals. An interesting fact that Joseph Pieper points out is that leisure in Greek is *skola* and in Latin, *scola*, the English 'school'. The word used to designate the place where we educate and teach is derived from a word which means 'leisure'. School does not, properly speaking, mean school, but 'leisure'. With the advances made in the modern age, the character and scope of education have changed; no longer does the formal academic curriculum dominate. Adult education, extension education and other similar forms of education thrive in an environment of rapid communication, which can teach and influence people in many kinds of situations and not simply in the classroom. Television, for example, can educate thousands of people about foreign affairs and vocational and cultural appreciation. The early pioneers of education, Froebel and Pestalozzi, stressed that the gap between play and learning in the development of young children and youth was mainly an adult conception and they contended that present day recreational pursuits and activities weaved in and out of the unstructured educational curriculum. It is a fact that students can learn readily and ably outside the classroom during playtime, which is their leisure time. This education sought during one's leisure could be labelled as an 'auxiliary curriculum'. Many educative acts may take place during a particular moment when people are completely unaware that such acts will have utility and purpose later. Some recreational activities are now accepted as part of the definition of the learning process. The question of how valid and reliable people should consider this interpretation may depend upon their own concept of education, its limitations, its expectations and its objectives.

Recreation and Physical Education

A common misconception is that recreation is synonymous with physical education. Too frequently, the belief is that since children play during the physical education period and on the playground after school hours, physical education and recreation are identical areas of endeavour. Such syllogistic reasoning disregards the distinctive characteristics of each field. In most states, physical education is an integral instructional part of the modern school curriculum. Educational law makes it compulsory for students to be taught physical education regularly by certified teachers. Physical education is often as much a required subject for graduation as history, English, mathematics and science. Instruction is devoted primarily to vigorous, 'big muscle' activities that are related to purposeful body movements, physical development and health. The curriculum is a series of progressive offerings for each grade from the elementary through the secondary levels, taking into consideration the needs, abilities and interests of the youth.

An important part of physical education is also related to hygienic care and community health problems. The recreational aspects of physical education may evolve directly or indirectly from regular instruction. One such example is intramural sport, which is the organization of students in the voluntary utilization of acquired athletic skills in regulated competition after the normal school day. Once students leave the classroom, it is quite natural that some of them will find use for the skills learned during the physical education period by using appropriate facilities in the community. It is a tribute to the dynamic nature of physical education and its teachers that such well taught skills are carried over into the everyday lives of students, many a time into the home environment. The value of physical education recreational skills has been substantiated by their place in different cultures, with athletics having emerged as a dominant part of many community recreation programmes.

Nevertheless, the distinction of recreation rests on its inclusiveness – its ability to include physical recreational aspects as well as activities of a social, cultural, aesthetic and mental nature. Recreation also symbolizes the theory that participation in leisure activities of an individual nature must rest upon the inviolate right of people to engage in such pursuits voluntarily. Re`creation presents the opportunities and experiences that people may enter into by means of what they may have acquired in their formal education, including physical education. Recreational experiences can be transformed and interpreted into personal values that make life more meaningful.

Recreation and Juvenile Delinquency

Is recreation the sole cure for juvenile delinquency? A popular view is: "To keep kids out of trouble, keep them busy." A ready solution, purportedly, is to provide youth with adequate playgrounds, offer an educational programme and, as a result, keep them from breaking the law. But society is now recognizing that recreation as a force in the community is but one of many factors to be considered in the assessment and prevention of juvenile delinquency. Recreational efforts have a contributing rather than a determining function in delinquency prevention. To fight juvenile delinquency adequately, it is logical and proper to consider and mobilize all community agencies and resources. Perhaps a most important consideration is that of parents and their task of providing decent homes and suitable family settings, though schools, social agencies, the police, courts and even industries can assist in the process. Many parts of the total community must be involved in a constructive effort to combat this evil, which has many complex aspects.

The misconception that recreation itself has the magical power to overcome delinquency rests upon a historical relationship. The early desire of the recreation leaders was to provide lay space for underprivileged children in crowded urban areas. It was believed that campaigns stressing the provision of recreational facilities would help the fight against crime and social ills. Such campaigns became popular and are still being perpetuated. Furthermore, welfare and health services in many communities tend to offer recreational services to youth as a part of their total programme. Since juvenile delinquency prevention is often stressed by such welfare agencies in their appeals for financial aid, recreation has been given a therapeutic connotation.

As a community force, recreation does have certain attributes, which can assist in the wide and varied fight against delinquency. Youth can be attracted and helped by proper recreational opportunities. The recreation centre can possess the facilities and leadership that will assist the potential delinquent or wayward youth to discover normal social behaviour. It would certainly not be irresponsible to conclude that the provision of regular recreational activities deters some youths from delinquency because they have ready access to enjoyable activities during their leisure time. It would also not be unreasonable to conclude that organized recreation will assume a delinquency prevention role if it makes a real effort to attract and hold youth, who would otherwise spend their leisure time wandering in search of 'something to do'.

We could make the further point that the development of recreational skills creates strong interests which allow no time for the kind of activities that lead youth into conflict with the law. But it is through integrated community efforts that recreational programmes can make their greatest contribution to prevent and curtail juvenile delinquency. Social problems are of such magnitude that they deserve expert attention and assistance from many quarters.

Recreational Needs and Children

Article 31 of the UN Convention on Child Rights states: "Every child has a right to rest and leisure, to engage in play and recreational activities appropriate to the age of the child and to participate freely in cultural life and the arts." However, fulfilment of this right is a dubious dream. We live in an examination conscious age, where children are often categorized on the basis of their academic performance. While seeking admission to highly competitive professional courses, the factor considered is a good academic performance. So children perceive examinations and results to be an indicator of their worth. Success in examinations is seen as a passport to a successful life and a determinant of a child's future. Failure in examinations is viewed as a catastrophe. It is no wonder that the very mention of examinations results in stress and psychiatric problems in children and disgust in parents. Confronted with the hopeless and frustrating examination process, many children find themselves under increasing stress. Sandwiched between an examination system that focuses on marks rather than achieving an ability to think and grow, many children of lower socio-economic status drop out. Stress builds as the level of education increases and by the time some of these children reach high school, they develop temperamental difficulties. In fact, children with temperamental dysfunctions, attention deficit disorders and conduct disorders are at higher risk of poor academic performance and emotional and behavioural disorders. Multiple retentions in the same grade are also a risk factor for further failures because failure begets failure. Parental pressure to perform is very high and, coupled with societal and peer pressures, an important cause of stress for children. External pressure only adds to self-created expectations and efforts to better one's own previous performance and this combined pressure occasionally becomes difficult for children to handle. Loss of self-esteem, a feeling of ineffectiveness, anxiety, depression and suicidal tendencies are seen before examinations. These emotional and behavioural disorders can be seen in some 20 per cent of schoolchildren. High parental aspirations and overt disappointment at a lower than expected performance lead to greater stress for children has shown that this is worse for girls. This could probably be because, in a male dominated society, female education is given low priority and girls are more likely to be pulled out of school if they perform poorly.

The problem of depression in teenagers and children is often hereditary in nature and, usually, it is those families that have a long history of depression that are the worst affected. Depressed children start withdrawing from daily activities. There is sudden change in appetite, leading to weight loss. They lack focus and concentration and show symptoms such as boredom, sadness, low self-esteem and self-destructive behaviour, leading ultimately to suicide. If you recognize these symptoms in a child around you, consult a doctor immediately because these indicate the initial stages of depression. A proper medical diagnosis is needed to discover the root cause of the problem. Depression and its symptoms can be alleviated with the help of medication, which includes natural remedies. You must remember that children are very sensitive and they cannot convey their feelings easily, so parents need to understand their children and give them proper medical care and recreation. According to different surveys, one out of every ten children suffers from feelings of depression. Feelings of depression, particular at a very young age, are extremely harmful. Reasons for depression among children, especially teenagers, are quite unpredictable. Teenage years in particular are sensitive for children and the problems faced by them at school and at home may lead to depression.

Benefits of Children Participating in Recreation

Children are always in a detention of sorts because their ability to engage in leisure activities and cultural life is automatically restricted.

For example, children cannot choose to go to a park or a cinema at will. They cannot decide whether or not to join the local football team or dance class. Recreation and participation in cultural life have a strong impact on children's development and mental health. Through play, children learn social and personal skills such as negotiation, sharing and self-control. For example, play can help child asylum seekers cope with what has happened to them, including past experiences of trauma and violence. Play relaxes children, relieves tensions, assists in the assimilation of learnt experiences, and helps them function better within the family and the community. Play and recreation can help them cope with all circumstances. Common elements such as celebrations of birthdays, arts and crafts classes, recreational videos after school and on weekends, organized sporting activities, supervised access to computers and excursions outside the school should be part of children's lives. Children's freedom to enjoy play and recreation is an important factor in determining what actions will be in their best interests. For example, the ability to play and participate in cultural life may affect a decision regarding whether or not to detain a child, where to detain a child or the conditions in which to detain a child.

Participation in recreational activities leads to well-balanced, healthy and physically active children. The early years are critical. Considerable evidence exists, which shows that the circumstances in the first years of children's lives have lifelong impacts on their health, learning and life skills. Recreation can play a positive role in their development. Participation in recreational programmes and activities benefits children in many ways:

- It promotes good physical and emotional development in them, helps them to develop motor skills, and stimulates their intellectual, emotional and social growth.
- It helps them to develop social skills, such as relating to others, learning social roles and reinforcing behavioural norms.
- It builds positive self-esteem and self-worth in them. Children gain a sense of achievement from mastering skills, which leads to higher achievement and better results in school.

- It develops life and leaderships skills in children by enabling them to participate in team and sports activities, become group leaders, make decisions and solve problems.
- It reduces the risk of diseases such as cardiovascular disease, cancer, diabetes, obesity and osteoporosis.
- It stimulates children's minds and creative thinking through play, games and creative programmes.
- It fosters an awareness of the larger community and cross-cultural understanding.
- It enables children with disorders to achieve the same level of social, physical and academic competencies as their peers
- It develops positive attitudes towards the importance of recreation and leisure in contributing to healthy, active lifestyles.
- It contributes to a healthier, stable family life when parents participate in their children's recreational activities.
- It provides fun, safe learning environments for children.
- Providing recreation for children is associated with good outcomes for mothers.

Children prefer to play games, rather than theoretical games. So include some educational games in the curriculum and use them to teach lessons; for example, tell a story with actions and, through the actions, introduce the names of animals and birds rather than just reading the story. Involve the children in the process. Other activities such as painting, dancing and singing can be included during the class schedule because such activities refresh the mind and children learn a lot from them. During after-school hours, hold classes for swimming and playing because these will offer children opportunities for entertainment and refreshment and also help in their physical development.

Do not force children to do any work or be involved in any activity. Let them choose the activity and then decide how you can relay an important message through that activity. For example, if a child likes to surf the Internet and to watch television, prepare video games that are both educative and recreational.

Intersperse activities such as games, singing and dancing along with other classes so that children do not feel bored with too much learning.

Organize weekly programmes so that students can take part in activities and competitions as they like, and offer prizes to attract them to participate. Celebrate all kinds of festivals in the school so that students realize that they are no different from the others and also learn more about different religions. Do not declare a holiday on a festival day; instead, encourage them to come to school and celebrate the festival with the other students and invite all the teachers and parents as well to participate in the celebrations.

Suggestions for Recreational Activities

The following activities are recreational when performed during leisure time, voluntarily, for the satisfaction inherent in them and for the socially accepted benefits they impart to the individual.

- *Arts and crafts:* These are activities, usually manual, such as drawing, modelling, painting, sculpting, sewing, photography, weaving and woodwork, which enable creative expression. Such creative activities enable individuals to express themselves freely. These self-determining acts translate ego centred involvement outward in the healthy process of self-realization. People are able to forget the normal restrictions of social customs and thereby answer a felt need for originality.
- *Music:* The effect that music has on individuals, whether as participants or as listeners, illustrates its unique attractions. Whether music is listened to for pure sensual pleasure, for aesthetic effect, for the rhythms produced, or whether people play or sing themselves, empathy and emotional release are generated quite obviously. There is hardly anyone who does not appreciate some form of music or the other.
- *Motor activities:* These include sports and exercise and serve to enhance physical vigour, improve physiological functioning, and sublimate socially disapproved feelings

through competitive experiences or individual acts in a social setting to provide satisfaction. Although many people take part in gross motor activities for achievement and self-realization, significant behaviour towards others is also developed. Activities include group and individual sports and games, team sports, and other competitive or non-competitive games.

- *Social activities:* Social needs are satisfied when people have to mix, get along or adjust with each other. Social activities of a wide scope have a place in any programme in which socially approved actions and good mental health are the objectives. The relationships developed through social intercourse contribute to the maturity of individuals, the development of empathy, sympathy, catharsis, personal esteem and self-expression.
- *Hobbies:* Hobbies are a stimulating and sustaining interest in an activity usually not connected with vocational experience. Hobbies include any human activity. Hobbies provide outlets for creative self-expression, self-determination and self-realization, and fulfil many needs in individuals because they come into contact with each another as they explore the manifestations of their particular interest.
- *Dance:* Dance is popular in its many forms because it deals with the universal and basic need for movement. It is a process of symbolic communication, expressing many sentiments as well as serving to fulfil emotional and physical feelings. It satisfies ambivalent desires and may be one method by which human beings satisfy hostility urges in socially acceptable ways.
- *Plays:* Plays are a form of communication through the human voice and body. As a communicative process, they offer satisfaction by transmitting ideas and emotions and providing self-expression either vicariously or directly. The elements of catharsis and empathy are closely related to dramatic reproductions.

- *Entertainment:* These are activities of a passive nature, such as television, radio, theatre or sports events, which engage people's attention in a satisfying manner.
- *Mental and literary activities*: These include reading, discussion groups, card games, public speaking, board games and writing and provide intellectual outlets and opportunities for creative expression.
- *Nature related activities:* These include camping, hiking, nature study and any activity that involves being in, using or interpreting the natural environment.
- *Special events:* These are organized activities that require special planning, as, for example, picnics, celebration of special days and holidays, festivals and fairs.
- *Sports, games and athletics:* These are activities involving gross physical movement such as organized informal games, as, for example, tag and relays, and individual, dual and team sports usually requiring facilities and equipment, such as track and field meets.
- *Social or civic services:* These include all the activities normally associated with altruistic or humanitarian programmes. Social service activities have long been utilized by recreationists to fill leisure productively; other forms of activity may not satisfy as well the human urge to extend sympathy or give aid. The release one obtains from wholeheartedly giving service to others and the exchange of too much self-concern for self-giving result in feelings of warm satisfaction.
- *Indoor activities:* Children should take part in indoor activities both to build their knowledge as well as for recreation. Such activities include playing indoor games, such as chess, Ludo, and other educational games.
- *Outdoor activities:* Children should take part in outdoor activities for their physical and mental fitness. These include games such as cricket, tennis, basketball and football.
- *Other activities:* Children should be socialized with other groups and they should make friends. Beside this, they should

focus on arts and crafts, painting and poetry, and develop hobbies.

Conclusion

Recreation and leisure services have a vital role to play in efforts to improve the lives of people living under adverse conditions. Recreation has a role in family, child and youth welfare; rural development; service to elderly people; the ailing; and other individuals in need of special attention. The emerging effort in recreation and leisure services is part of a larger effort in the nation through education, employment, health and social welfare. Recreation is for everyone, regardless of occupation, age, race, income or any other factor. Everyone needs some relaxation and refreshment. People in a community participate in a recreational programme as members of the community, not as employees of a particular factory, group or nationality. An important point here is that children, women and elderly people are the most vulnerable groups and they are unable to take part in many regular recreational activities.

Bibliography

Abrahamsen, David. 1999. *The Psychology of Crime*. Columbia University Press, New York.

Aichhorn, A. 1989. *Delinquency and Child Guidance*. International University Press, New York.

Alure, M. 2002. *Invisible Children: A Study of Policy Exclusion*. Viva Books New Delhi Pvt. Ltd., New Delhi.

Andry, R.G. 2002. *Delinquency and Parental Pathology*. Methuen & Co. Ltd., London.

Bharadhwaj, R.K. 1992. *Urban Development in India*. National Publication House, New Delhi.

Butler, G. 1976. *Introduction to Community Recreation*. McGraw Hill Book Co., New York.

Josvaha, T. 1994. *Recreation and Leisure for Children*. Thomas Press, New Zealand. Wellington.

Kraus, R. 1964. *Recreation and the Schools*. Macmillan Co., New York.

Kundu, C.L. 1997. *Personality Development: A Critique of Indian Studies*. Vishal Publications, Rohtak.

Muraldharan, R. and Asthana, S. 1991. *Stimulation Activities for Young Children: A Model for Parents and Child Care Workers*. National Council for Educational Research and Training, New Delhi.

Rende, R.D. and Plomin, R. 1992. 'Relations between First Grade Stress, Temperament and Behaviour Problems'. *Journal of Maharashtra Agricultural University*, 13: pp. 435–46.

10 Health Education in Schools

The Portuguese brought tobacco to India in the beginning of the 17th century. The higher echelons of Indian society first enjoyed the pleasures of tobacco during the rule of the Mughal king, Jehangir. Slowly, tobacco trickled down to the common people. It was a novelty at first, but soon became a craving among people of all classes of society, permeating even villages. Addictions developed over time. As its use became widespread, farming of tobacco was started. The soil and climate of India were favourable to tobacco farming and tobacco was soon recognized as a high income yielding crop. Tobacco farming first started in Gujarat and Maharashtra and then spread to other regions. Even today, tobacco farming takes place on a large scale in Gujarat. As tobacco is dangerous to human health, the government has imposed several restrictions on tobacco production. Today, people in villages smoke bidis, hookahs or pipes. School-children smoke bidis and eat *gutka.* Young educated and rich people smoke cigarettes.

Tobacco is consumed mainly in two forms – chewing and smoking – and it is the main reason for oral cancer: Around 90 per cent of oral cancers in Southeast Asia are linked to tobacco chewing and tobacco smoking. Oral cancers are mainly attributed to tobacco chewing. In developing countries, 2–10 per cent women and 40–60 per cent men use tobacco. Tobacco use usually begins in adolescence – the time for discovery, challenge and experimentation. Children receive tobacco from their parents, especially women, right from their childhood.

Table 10.1 *Preferred Places for Purchase of Gutka*

Place	*School Students*	*Percentage (%)*
School Premises	30	24.0
Shops Near School	57	45.6
Shops Near Home	09	7.2
Shops on Way to School	29	23.2
Total	125	100.0

Source: Pawar, A.B., and Mukherjee, S. 2004–07. 'Gutkha and Tobacco Consumption and Awareness of Their Health Hazards among School Students in Gujarat, in India' in *Journal of Community Medicine*, Vol. 29, No. 3.

The figures in Table 10.1 clearly indicate that students prefer *paan* shops on the way to school and around the school premises for the purchase of tobacco products because such shops are far away from their homes and they need not fear being caught by their parents.

Primary prevention of tobacco can be implemented in the form of a community approach, in which the risk of the entire community is eliminated without the individual's direct participation. Some of these measures include higher taxation on tobacco and tobacco products, changes in the manufacturing process of tobacco products, ban on tobacco sale, alternative crops for tobacco farmers, etc. Recently, the Maharashtra, Uttar Pradesh and Rajasthan governments have imposed a ban on the production and sale of *gutka* in these states. This could be a major milestone in tobacco control, if implemented properly.

Smoking Tobacco

Tobacco smoke contains nicotine, an addictive stimulant. The effect of nicotine in first time or irregular users is an increase in alertness and memory and mild euphoria. In chronic users, nicotine simply relieves the symptoms of nicotine withdrawal: confusion, restlessness, anxiety, insomnia and dysphasia. Nicotine also disturbs the metabolism and suppresses the appetite. This is because nicotine, like many stimulants, increases blood sugar.

Chewing Tobacco

You may hear more about the harm cigarettes do to the body, but chewing tobacco is just as harmful. Chewing tobacco can cause sores and white patches in the mouth, leading to diseases and cancers of the mouth, gums and throat. Chewing can result in bad breath, discolouration of the teeth and tooth loss. One chew of tobacco contains 15 times the nicotine in a cigarette, which means that the risk of addiction is much higher. The tobacco in cigarettes also contains nicotine, the substance that makes smoking addictive. All of these things are bad for the human body. Nicotine raises risk of heart attacks and strokes. Tobacco is toxic to the body. It causes more health problems and early deaths than all the illegal drugs combined. On top of that, tobacco is addictive. This means that once people start using it, their bodies get addicted to it. Everyone who smokes starts by 'just trying it'. That is how the habit and the addiction begin.

Methods of Smoking

Cigarettes

Cigarette smoking is the most common form of tobacco consumption. A cigarette is a product manufactured from cured and cut tobacco leaves, which are rolled and/or stuffed into a paper wrapped cylinder. Because of the curing process, the smoke is mild enough to inhale in large quantities, unlike cigar or pipe tobacco.

Cigars

A cigar is a cylinder of tobacco rolled in tobacco leaves, which is generally puffed at, not inhaled. Cigars come in many shapes and sizes, the most common being Corona, Cigarillo and Robusto. Cigars generally come in two colours, 'natural' and 'Maduro'.

Pipes

A tobacco pipe typically consists of a small chamber (bowl) for the combustion of the substance to be smoked and a thin stem (shank) that ends in a mouthpiece (also called a 'bit'). Pipes are made from a variety of materials – briar, corncob, meerschaum, clay, wood, glass, gourd, bamboo and metal. Tobacco pipes are often chemically treated to change the smell and taste of tobacco; other commercially available tobacco products do not have this feature. Younger and middle aged smokers, hit by the onslaught of cigarette advertising, find the tobacco pipe's contemplative nature and age transcendent status 'a hobby, not a habit', which is both thoroughly enjoyable and stress relieving.

Hookahs

Hookahs (or sheeshas) are traditional West Asian and South Asian water pipes, which operate through water filtration and indirect heat. Hookahs are very popular in West Asia, but form a niche market in many other parts of the world as well. Some flavours of tobacco used in hookahs are the traditional apple, grape, orange, strawberry, cherry, mango, vanilla and melon and the more modern cola, coconut, cappuccino, and banana milk. In other contexts, hookahs are used to smoke cannabis, hashish or opium.

Snuff

Snuff is a generic term for fine-ground, smokeless tobacco products. Originally, the term referred only to dry snuff, a fine tan dust popular mainly in the 18th century. This was also called Scotch Snuff, a folk etymology derivation of the scorching process used to dry cured tobacco in the factory. Snuff powder originated in the UK town of Great Harwood and was famously ground there prior to local distribution. Snuff has been found to be beneficial in some cases of hay fever due to the fact that it may prevent allergens from getting to the mucus membrane in the nose.

Chewing Tobacco

Chewing is one of the oldest ways of consuming tobacco leaves.

Suns

The Swedish *suns* is made from steam cured tobacco, not fire cured tobacco, and its health effects are markedly different, with epidemiological studies showing lower rates of cancer and other tobacco related health problems than cigarettes.

Gutka

Gutka (also spelt as *gutkha*, *guttkha* or *guthka*) is a preparation of crushed betel nuts, tobacco, and sweet or savoury flavourings. It is manufactured in India and exported to a few other countries. A mild stimulant, it is sold across India in small, individual size packets. It is consumed much like chewing tobacco and, like chewing tobacco, it is considered responsible for oral cancer and other severe negative health effects. Used by millions of adults, it is also marketed to children. Some packaging does not mention tobacco as an ingredient and some brands are pitched as candy – featuring brightly coloured packaging with children's faces. Some are chocolate flavoured and some are marketed as breath fresheners.

Tobacco Water

Tobacco water is a traditional organic insecticide used in domestic gardening. Tobacco dust can be used similarly. Tobacco water is produced by boiling strong tobacco in water or by steeping tobacco in water for a longer period. When cooled, the mixture can be applied as a spray or 'painted' onto the leaves of garden plants, where it acts as an insecticide.

Why People are Attracted to Tobacco

Advertising

Before the 1970s, most tobacco advertising was legal. Tobacco smoking is still advertized in special magazines, during sporting events, in gas stations and stores and, in more rare cases, on television. Some nations, including the UK and Australia, have begun anti-smoking advertisements to counter the effects of tobacco advertising. The actual effectiveness of tobacco advertising is widely documented. According to an opinion piece by Henry Saffer, public health experts say that tobacco advertising increases cigarette consumption and there is much empirical literature that indicates a significant effect of tobacco advertising on smoking, especially among children.

Peer Pressure

Many anti-smoking organizations claim that teenagers begin smoking because of peer pressure and the cultural influences portrayed by friends. However, it is found that direct pressure to smoke cigarettes plays a significant part in adolescent smoking. Adolescents have reported high levels of both normative and direct pressure to smoke cigarettes.

Parental Smoking

Children of parents who smoke are more likely to take up cigarettes than children of parents who do not. It is found that parental cigarette addiction was associated with less adolescent smoking, except when the other parent continued to smoke. Different studies tested the relationship between adolescent smoking and rules regulating where adults were allowed to smoke in the home. Results showed that restrictive home smoking policies were associated with lower likelihood of trying smoking among both middle and high school students.

Smoking in Movies and TV Programmes

Exposure to smoking in movies has been linked with adolescent smoking initiation in several cross-sectional studies. Films tend to have a high incidence of smoking behaviour vis-à-vis the general population. According to a study of movies created between 1988 and 1997, 87 per cent of these movies portrayed various kinds of tobacco use, with an average of five occurrences per film. R-rated movies had the greatest number of such occurrences and were most likely to feature major characters using tobacco. There have been moves to reduce the depiction of protagonists smoking in television shows, especially those aimed at children.

Ill-Effects of Tobacco

Mouth, Throat and Oesophagus

Smoking is a risk factor for cancers of the larynx, oral cavity and oesophagus. More than 90 per cent of patients with oral cancer (including cancers of the lip, tongue, mouth and throat) are found to be smokers and the risk for these cancers increases with the number of cigarettes smoked. Heavy smokers have laryngeal cancer mortality risks 20–30 times greater than non-smokers. The combined effect of tobacco increases the risk of oral and pharyngeal cancers 35-fold.

Heart and Circulation

Two immediate effects of smoking on the heart and circulation are an increase in the heartbeat rate and a sharp rise in blood pressure. These responses are caused by nicotine, which acts on the nervous system, causing the heart rate to rise and blood vessels to constrict. This narrowing of the blood vessels causes blood pressure rise and the heart to come under strain. The carbon monoxide in cigarettes depletes the oxygen carrying capacity of a smoker's blood. This means that the heart has to pump harder to get enough oxygen to the rest of the body.

Lungs

The tar content of cigarette smoke damages the cells in the airways of the lungs, rendering the cilia unable to sweep away the harmful substances. Eventually, this damage can produce cells that grow in an uncontrolled way, leading to cancer of the lungs or larynx. Moreover, harmful substances from the smoke are detected by the protective cells of the body and these cells move to the lungs and try to defend them, but are destroyed by the cigarette smoke. The dead cells release substances that damage the structure of the lungs, leading to chronic bronchitis and emphysema. Tobacco accounts for more than 80 per cent of lung cancer cases. The observed relationship between tobacco smoking and the incidence of lung cancer appears to depend on factors such as the daily dose of tobacco; the duration of regular smoking; and the form in which the tobacco is smoked (cigarettes, cigars, pipes).

Brain

Cigarette smoking has been linked to the build-up of fatty substances in the carotid artery, the main neck artery supplying blood to the brain. Blockage of this artery may cut off the blood supply to the brain cells, which results in strokes (cerebral thrombosis). Also, nicotine raises blood pressure; carbon monoxide reduces the amount of oxygen your blood can carry to the brain; and cigarette smoke makes the blood thicker and more likely to clot. Smokers are more likely to have a stroke than non-smokers, with the overall relative risk of a stroke in smokers being about 1.5 times that in non-smokers.

Digestive System

Smoking has been shown to have harmful effects on all parts of the digestive system, contributing to such common disorders as heartburn and peptic ulcers. It also increases the risk of Crohn's disease and possibly gallstones. Risk of stomach cancer caused by smoking increases with the duration of smoking and the number of cigarettes smoked.

Liver and Pancreas

Nearly 50 per cent of bladder and kidney cancers in men are caused by smoking, with a lower contribution in women. Cigarette smoke can interact with chemicals (especially aromatic amines) in the workplace to produce bladder and kidney cancer. Also, around 30 per cent of all deaths from pancreatic cancer are attributable to cigarette smoking.

Skin and Hair

Just 10 minutes of cigarette smoking decreases the body's and skin's oxygen supply for almost an hour. Smoking robs the skin of collagen, which keeps it elastic. Smokers get more and deeper wrinkles all over their faces because nicotine constricts the tiny capillaries that nourish the skin. Smokers in their 40s often have as many facial wrinkles as non-smokers in their 60s. Smoking interferes with the healing process – it takes longer to heal and there is more scarring. Smokers are also prone to premature thinning and greying of the hair. Men who smoke are twice as likely to become bald as are men who smoke, and premature greying is three-six times more common in smokers.

Bones and Muscles

Smoking delays the healing of fractures, and in some smokers, bone healing is indefinitely delayed. Nicotine restricts blood flow to all tissue, especially in the newly forming tissues that are involved in bone repair. Moreover, tobacco smoke contains poisonous chemicals that inhibit the development of new tissue cells. Smokers' tissues do not get adequate blood supply to promote healing, so they are at a much higher risk of developing osteoporosis. Male smokers are also affected because smoking affects the production of bone cells negatively.

Justification for the Project

The Department of Extension and Communication, Faculty of Family and Community Sciences, MS University of Baroda, in Vadodara, has undertaken various action projects covering thrust areas such as environment education, income generating activities and health. The Department has also undertaken various activities related to health issues such as plays, expert talks and experiments with educational games. Several research studies and surveys on health issues have been conducted on topics such as the nutritional status of the girl child in the family, assessment of the health and nutritional status of underprivileged school age boys and reproductive health of women. Similarly, the Department has conducted projects such as starting eco clubs, literacy through games, and training women to start day care centres. In the field of health, different action projects have been conducted on topics such as reproductive health and HIV/AIDS, but no action project has been taken up on the prevention of tobacco use or providing education on tobacco control. Thus, keeping in mind the important issue of health, the Department's project workers planned to offer awareness about tobacco control in a school in Vadodara city.

Tobacco chewing exists in one form or the other almost everywhere in India and it has become a serious social and health problem. The reasons why people take on this habit vary not only on account of individual and social differences, but also because of other uncertain factors, such as the economic, physical, mental and cultural status of the individual. The more serious and dangerous aspect of the problem is that people across social strata are becoming increasingly addicted to tobacco. There is growing concern about this because of the likelihood of its further increase, especially in slums and rural areas.

We live in an examination conscious age where children are often categorized on the basis of their academic performance. While seeking admission to highly competitive professional courses, the vital factor is a good academic performance. So children perceive examinations and their results to be an indicator of their worth. Success in examinations is seen as a passport to a successful life and the determinant of the future of children. Confronted with a hopeless and frustrating examination process, many children find themselves under increasing stress, Sandwiched between an examination system that focuses on marks rather than achieving an ability to think and grow, many children from the lower socio-economic strata drop out. Stress builds as the level of education increases and, by the time some of these children reach high school, they develop temperamental difficulties. In fact, children with temperamental dysfunctions, attention deficit disorders and conduct disorders are at higher risk of poor academic performance and emotional and behavioural disorders. Multiple retentions in the same grade are a risk factor for further failures. Parental pressure to perform is very high as are societal and peer pressures. All these induce stress in children. External pressure only adds to their self-created expectations and efforts to better previous performances and this combined pressure occasionally becomes difficult for children to handle. Loss of self-esteem, a feeling of ineffectiveness, anxiety, depression and suicidal tendencies are seen before examinations. These emotional and behavioural disorders can be seen in up to 20 per cent of schoolchildren (*Times of India*, November 2007).

The problem of depression in teenagers and children is often due to hereditary reasons and families that have a long history of depression are usually the worst affected. It must be remembered that children are very sensitive and cannot convey their feelings easily, so parents need to understand their children and give them proper medical care and recreation. According to a survey, one out of every ten children suffers from feelings of depression. Depression at such a young age can be very harmful. Depressed children start withdrawing from their daily activities and exhibit symptoms such as boredom, sadness and low self-esteem. If you notice such symptoms in a child around you, consult a doctor immediately as these signs indicate the start of depression. Teenage years are sensitive years for children and the reasons for depression among them vary. Lack of self-expression and feelings of disgust lead children towards addictions and self-destructive behaviour.

The project took up for its focus the Class VII students of a municipal school in Vadodara city. This particular class was chosen because the children were at an age when they should learn about the harmful effects of tobacco use. Schools are important for the cognitive, creative and social development of children. Tobacco use has been suggested as an important risk factor of overall concern.

The use of tobacco is harmful to general health and is a common cause of addiction, illness, disability and death. The use of tobacco leads to an increased risk of oral cancer, periodontal disease, oral mucosal lesions and other deleterious oral conditions and it adversely affects the outcome of rural health. It has been scientifically proven that tobacco causes more than 20 categories of fatal and disabling disease, including cancer, cardiovascular disease and chronic respiratory disease. Use of tobacco currently accounts for three million deaths each year worldwide and nearly a third of these deaths occur in India alone. These facts acted as an imperative for the project.

Objectives of the Project

- To impart education on tobacco control to the Class VII students of Municipal School No. 14, Opposite S.R. Petrol Pump, Nizampura, Vadodara
- To make the students aware of the ill-effects of tobacco chewing.
- To involve them in organizing various activities related to tobacco control.
- To evaluate their awareness and understanding of concepts related to tobacco control.

Methodology

To make any programme effective and successful, the very first step is the drawing up of a plan of the action. Systematic planning can provide the necessary guidelines to implement the programme successfully. Planning indicates focus and gives priority and design for the work. Planning is required to carry out the work successfully and smoothly.

Planning for the Project

To start the project, systematic planning was done as follows:

Identifying the School

Three schools were contacted to impart tobacco education: Municipal School No. 6, Behind Rangoli Restaurant, Fatehgunj; Municipal School No. 14, Opposite S.R. Petrol Pump, Nizampura, Vadodara; and Rosary School, Pratapgunj, Vadodara. The principals of these schools were given an orientation in the project. Two schools did not show any interest and declined to hold such activities in their schools because of their fixed academic schedules. The principal of Municipal School No. 14 showed an interest in starting the project in his school.

Deciding the Venue and Time for the Project

A meeting was held with the administrative staff and the principal of the school to decide the venue, class, timing, teacher and coordinator for the activities. The school authority allotted four days – Monday, Tuesday, Wednesday and Saturday – from 3 pm to 5 pm for the project activities. The venue for all the activities was the students' classroom. It was also decided at the meeting that the students of Class VII were the most suitable for this project because they were not overburdened academically and were mature enough to understand the problem of tobacco chewing.

Contacting the Students

The students of Class VII were contacted for the project and their interest in such activities was assessed. Finally, they were oriented in the tobacco education that was to be imparted in the school with their help. Several visits were made to the school to build a rapport with the children.

Obtaining Permission from the Shikshan Adhikari Samiti

Written permission from the Shikshan Adhikari Samiti to conduct the action project on tobacco control at Municipal School No. 14 was obtained before starting the project.

Contacting Resource Persons

Resource persons were contacted for their help and guidance in imparting education on tobacco control and to conduct activities such as a movie on tobacco and expert talks.

Table 10.2 *List of Experts Involved in the Project*

Topic	*Resource Person*
Expert Talk on ill effect of tobacco chewing	Anand Bhai, Administrator, Kripa, an NGO working on tobacco control
Expert Talk on Tobacco Control	Yogesh Patel, Nizampura, Vadodara
Yoga	Dushyant Shah, Arvind Ashram, Dandiya Bazar, Vadodara
Health Check-Up	Hasmukh M. Shah, Sultanpura, Vadodara

Selection of the Content

The selection of the content for the project activities was done by referring to books and a list of activities. The project worker talked to the experts regarding the project and its importance, its objectives and its advantages. Handouts were prepared for reference. The different topics that were covered were:

- Importance of health.
- Types of addiction.
- Recreational activities.
- Harmful effects of tobacco chewing.
- Different types of diseases caused by tobacco chewing.

Preparing Teaching Aids

Teaching aids help learners to understand concepts more easily. Several experiments have shown that teaching aids can be helpful in making any programme successful. The project worker prepared and borrowed teaching aids that were suitable for particular activities under the project.

Table 10.3 *Different Types of Teaching Aids Used*

Teaching Aids	*Topics*
Posters	Illustrative talk on how tobacco affects health
Flash Cards	Methods of tobacco consumption
Charts, Banners, Posters	Campaign
Specimens	Story on tobacco chewing
Mobiles	Motivational activities
Puppets	Play
Models	Illustrative talk
Handouts	Illustrative talk
Educational Games	Snakes and Ladders Puzzle game
Flip Charts	Summarization

Schedule of Activities

To impart education and to create awareness about tobacco use, different activities were planned:

Expert talk	Yoga
Health check-ups	Film show
Educational game	Motivational activities
Drawing competition	Essay competition
Illustrative talk	Play
Campaigning	Exhibition
Role play	

Activities Conducted under the Project

The details of the activities conducted under the project are given here:

Orientation

Objective: To orient the students regarding the project.

Activity: The project worker oriented the students with the help of the teacher and the coordinator on what tobacco was and the activities related to tobacco control. She also talked about what tobacco control was and the importance of health care.

Illustrative Talk

Objective: To create awareness regarding the effects of tobacco amongst the students.

Activity: First, the project worker explained what tobacco was and the different methods of consuming it. She then gave an illustrative talk on the effects of tobacco consumption, using posters and flip charts to make her talk easier to understand. After finishing the talk, she summarized what she had told them with the help of flip charts.

Gain: The students gained knowledge about the ill effects of chewing tobacco.

Expert Talk

Objective: To orient the students on how to quit tobacco chewing.

Activity: Mr Anand Patel, Administrator of Kripa, a non-governmental organization (NGO) working on tobacco control, was invited to give the expert talk. Mr Patel explained the different methods and steps to quit tobacco chewing. He told the students about the disadvantages of tobacco and its bad effect on health. The talk was concluded with a discussion.

Gain: The students became aware of the importance of health and the bad effects of tobacco on the human body.

Drawing Competition

Objective: To enhance the students' creativity.

Activity: The project worker asked the students to draw a picture of the harmful effects of tobacco and the different methods of tobacco consumption. She then asked them to come up with slogans for stopping tobacco use. She provided drawing sheets and colouring materials. The students had to come up with pictures in an hour. At the end of the time, the project worker announced two winners of the competition and gave them motivational gifts.

Gain: Novel and creative ideas were gathered by the project, which further helped in its development.

Role Play

Objective: To motivate the students to participate in role play.

Activity: In this activity, the students had to perform different roles. The project worker gave them different situations and some time for rehearsal. After that, the students performed their derivation of the situations.

Gain: The students learned to speak in front of the public about situations related to tobacco consumption that they encounter at home or in public places.

Game

Objective: To motivate the students to adopt good habits.

Activity: The project worker borrowed a Snakes and Ladders game from the Department of Extension and Communication. She formed different questions related to education. Then she gave instructions on how to play the game and its rules and regulations. Initially, six students started to play; when any of the playing members won and got out of the game, new members were added.

Gain: The students got to know that if they followed good habits in their lives as given in the game, they would enjoy good health and be winners in life.

Film Show

Objective: To help the students understand better the harmful effects of tobacco.

Activity: The project worker got a film, *Issues on Tobacco*, from Kripa. She arranged for a television set and a DVD player. The film was in Gujarati, so the students could understand it quite easily. The film was around 45 minutes long and it covered issues related to the effects of tobacco. The students enjoyed it.

Gain: The students were made aware of the effects of tobacco chewing.

Educational Game

Objective: To encourage the students to take active part in the educational games on 'Tabacco'.

Activity: Two types of games were played by the participants. The first was a 'join the parts' game. The students had to join different parts of a picture and make a whole one; the picture was related to tobacco use. This game was played in small groups.

The second was a musical game. The students had to pass through different squares with music playing. When the music stopped, each student had to pick up a slip of paper from wherever he/she had landed and answer the question on the slip of paper.

The project worker gave the instructions for both games before they were played. The students said they liked both games very much.

Gain: The students got confidence in giving answers.

Essay Competition

Objective: To improve the students' knowledge regarding different topics of tobacco chewing.

Activity: The project worker gave instructions to the students on how to write an essay and what kind of sub-topics they should cover. The students were given an hour to write their essays. The project worker then checked all the essays and announced three winners. She gave motivational gifts to the winners.

Gain: The students learned to express their thoughts and this raised their confidence levels.

Play

Objective: To explain to the students the practical effects of tobacco chewing.

Activity: A highly motivational play, on the topic of tobacco control, was performed by the third year students of Home Science Extension and Communication. It was liked by the students. Once the play was over, the project worker discussed the merits and demerits of tobacco chewing with the students.

Gain: It was concluded that a play was the best way of imparting knowledge about the harmful effects of tobacco chewing to the students.

Motivational Activity

Objective: To built a rapport with the students.

Activity: The project worker involved the students in many motivational activities, such as games, songs, and art and craft, which they enjoyed thoroughly. Thus, the project worker motivated the students, developed their creative skills and built a rapport with them.

Campaign

Objective: To create awareness regarding tobacco control amongst all primary school children.

Activity: Students of the primary section of the school took part in the campaigning. They used different teaching materials like charts, posters and banners to create awareness among the other students of the school. They enjoyed it very much. The slogans were repeated by the students. The project worker told the students about the merits of campaigning.

Gain: Students who are involved in such activities gain knowledge and students who are not involved also get information about tobacco.

Exhibition

Objective: To develop exhibition organizing skills amongst the students.

Activity: At the end of the project, the project worker, with the help of the students, prepared an exhibition. All the teaching aids, such as charts and posters, were exhibited. The charts and posters were explained by the students to other students. The effect of this exhibition was widespread.

Gain: The students got a good chance to explore their abilities, skills and creativity.

Evaluation of the Project

The word 'evaluation', comes from the Latin word, 'valere', meaning strong or valiant. Its dictionary meaning is the determination of value, the strength or worth of something, an appraisal, an estimate of the force or making of judgement of something. Evaluation in general refers to appraisal, determining the strength and weakness or success and failure of a programme. Evaluation depends upon measurement, but is not synonymous with measurement. Evaluation goes beyond measurement or answering the question whether the obtained measurement is desirable or undesirable. Evaluation is useful in revealing the stage at which the target group has arrived at a learning process. As we all know, extension education forms a live contact between knowledge sources (institutions) and social situations (communities) by way of addressing the latter's problems and issues. As people have different interests and needs, extension education has to be broad and varied in its meaning to meet the interests of the people it serves. The idea behind the tobacco control education project was to develop the social behaviour of the beneficiaries, which would, in turn, bring about a change in their different groups and the intra- and inter-relationships of the social groups. The topic of tobacco control is an important issue for proper development and the students were taught and trained so that the developmental communication messages spread across the community. To check the effectiveness of the project, the project worker evaluated it.

Evaluation of the Project on the Basis of the Rating Scale Background Information

Table 10.4 *Percentage Distribution of Class VII Students According to Age*

(N = 35)

Age in Years	*Frequency (f)*	*Percentage (%)*
11	5	14.29
12	10	28.57
13	10	28.57
14	10	28.57

Table 10.4 indicates that the majority of the respondents were 12–14 years old.

Table 10.5 *Percentage Distribution of Class VII Students According to Father's Occupation*

(N = 35)

Occupation of Father	*Frequency (f)*	*Percentage (%)*
Sweeper	10	28.57
Rickshaw Driver	10	28.57
Job	15	42.86

Table 10.5 indicates that a large majority of the students' fathers were holding a job and the majority of the students' fathers were rickshaw drivers or sweepers.

Table 10.6 *Percentage Distribution of Class VII Students According to Mother's Occupation*

(N = 35)

Occupation of Mother	*Frequency (f)*	*Percentage (%)*
Housewife	25	71.43
Part-time servants	10	28.57

Table 10.6 indicates that a large majority of the students' mothers were engaged in household activities as housewives, whereas the remaining students' mothers were engaged as part-time servants in nearby colonies. It is clear from Tables 10.4 and 10.5 that the children in Municipal School No. 14 belong to a low socio-economic background: This is evident from the occupations of both their mothers and their fathers.

Table 10.7 *Percentage Distribution of Class VII Students According to their Attendance in Project Activities*

(N = 35)

Attendance	*Yes (%)*	*No (%)*
Attended all the activities	85	15

Table 10.7 indicates that a large majority of the students – 85 per cent – could attend all the project activities, and only around 15 per cent students were unable to do so.

Table 10.8 *Percentage Distribution Class VII Students According to Reasons for Not Attending Project Activities*

(N = 6)

Reasons for Not Attending All the Project Activities	*Yes (%)*
Was not well	14.28
Had gone out of town	8.57

Table 10.8 indicates that 14.28 per cent of the students could not attend all the project activities because they were not well and 8.57 per cent of the students could not attend them because they had gone out of town.

Table 10.9 *Percentage Distribution of Class VII Students According to their Interest in the Various Project Activities*

(N = 35)

Activities	*Interesting*	*Less Interesting*
Drawing Competition	84.35	15.65
Expert Talk	91.11	8.89
Games	100.00	—
Role Play	93.78	6.22
Play	97.78	2.22
Yoga	82.29	17.71
Film Show	100.00	—
Essay Competition	76.59	23.41
Exhibition	98.87	1.13
Demonstration of open stand	90.18	9.82

Table 10.9 indicates that all the students of Class VII – 100 per cent – found the educational games and movie very interesting. A very large majority of the students – 98.87 per cent – found the exhibition and play interesting. A majority of the students found the drawing competition, expert talk, role play, Yoga and demonstration of pen stand interesting. Only 76.59 per cent of the students found the essay competition interesting. The reason for this could be that teaching aids are defined as materials that communicate facts and ideas clearly through a combination of words and pictures. The project worker visited different organizations to collect teaching aids such as charts and posters and prepared different kinds of teaching aids for clarity on the topics, subjects and activities that were taken up. Teaching aids such as charts, posters, flash cards, flip charts and specimens were used. These teaching aids must have played a vital role in making the education a reality for the students because they help in learning and understanding knowledge quickly.

The project worker purposely selected different teaching aids and teaching methods so that they maximized the learning and made it easy for the students to grasp and retain the verbal explanation of the topic, 'Tobacco', which was otherwise very abstract. The teaching aids helped to create a dynamic learning environment by shifting emphasis from the spoken word to an instructional methodology. The project worker wanted to ensure that everything she taught the students during the project on tobacco control had a lasting effect on their minds. She took immense care while selecting the teaching aids, which proved to be excellent for the individual approach and for the group approach. All the teaching aids were prepared by the project worker according to the content and relevance of the activities conducted. Each topic was explained in detail with the help of charts and posters; for more clarity, specimens, mobiles and samples were also displayed.

Table 10.10 *Percentage Distribution of Class VII Students According to the Effectiveness of the Various Project Activities*

(N = 35)

Activities	*Great Extent (%)*	*Less Extent (%)*
Expert talk about tobacco related diseases	91.11	8.89
Play	97.31	2.69
Educational game	100.00	–

Table 10.10 indicates that all the students found the educational game – 100 per cent – and play – 97.31 per cent – the most effective method to convey the message against tobacco use. A very large majority of the students – 91.11 per cent – found the expert talk and the importance of health most effective. A game is an educational play situation possessing some structure by virtue of a set of rules or procedures to be followed. Games may require varying degrees of skill, concentration and coordination, depending upon their organization and execution. With games such as these, play has to be finished before the discussion can start, so timing is important. 'What do I want my students to learn from playing this?' is of prime importance.

The word 'game', comes from the old Teutonic word meaning joy. It denotes an activity indulged in and for the sake of the pleasure it gives, rather than any other purpose. It denotes, in a narrower sense, a contest carried out according to rules and decided by the strength, skill or luck of the contestants. Games are a natural and essential element of human development. They are an important method by which people are provided knowledge, experience and entertainment. The interest in games is a complex of instinctive tendencies, which is a striking feature of human nature, not only of children, but also of adults across social strata.

Table 10.10 further shows that plays were found to be a very effective medium for communicating the message against tobacco use. Whether one acts or observes, dramatization is a substitute for the real experience. The experience is, of course, much more immediate and meaningful to the one who plays a part in the play than to someone who merely watches. Dramatic participation and dramatic observation are two faces of the same coin. Plays can do more than teach important ideas to participants and observers of all ages. They can also pose new questions for them to think about. Thus, plays start currents in the minds of the participants and the audience. This could have been the reason why a large majority of the students liked the play.

Table 10.11 *Percentage Distribution of Class VII Students According to Changes Adopted after Getting the Information about Tobacco*

(N = 35)

Changes Adopted	*Great Extent (%)*	*Less Extent (%)*
Now I do not chewing gutka or tobacco	93.18	6.82
I have stopped keeping in touch with people who chewing gutka or tobacco	77.78	22.22
I also prevent my friends chewing gutka or tobacco	95.56	4.41
I am ready to take part in all tobacco control activities	98.20	1.80

Table 10.11 indicates that a very large majority of the students reported that they no longer consume *gutka* or tobacco. They prevent their friends from consuming tobacco products. They are ready to take part in all anti-tobacco activities. A large section of the

students even stopped fraternizing with students who were consuming *gutka* or tobacco.

Table 10.12 *Percentage Distribution of Class VII Students in Relation to Taking Part in Future Tobacco Control Activities*

(N = 35)

Future Actions	*Yes (%)*
Ready to take part in tobacco control activities in the future	100
Motivate other students to join in tobacco control activities	100
Every school should have tobacco control activities	100

Table 10.12 indicates that all the students agreed to participate in future tobacco control activities and they felt that every school should get information on tobacco control. The table also shows that all the students reported that they would like to motivate others to join similar tobacco control activities.

Indications of increasing tobacco use among children are a matter of concern. The Tobacco Control Act, which was passed in 2003, is a milestone and the need of the hour is effective enforcement of the law. Till now, schools had monitors to mind discipline in class. But with nearly one in every ten school children, aged 13–15, consuming some form of tobacco, the Union Ministry of Health is now planning to introduce a new kind of classroom enforcer – the tobacco monitor. Part of the strategy is to involve youth in the fight against tobacco, so these monitors will not only act as peer educators to deter their classmates from smoking, but will also have the power to check bags for tobacco products.

Tobacco education is also being made part of the school curriculum to make students aware of the bad effects of smoking. Each school has been allocated by state government around Rs 8,000 for conducting anti-tobacco activities. According to the plan, more than 50 schools in each district are part of the pilot project. Students are being sensitized so that they became the anti-tobacco ambassadors of the future. Schools in Gujarat already have tobacco monitors who are authorized to go through their schoolmates' bags for tobacco products. The plan is to have 30–40 high school students in every school trained as monitors, who will also act as peer educators to deter classmates from consuming tobacco products, both within and outside school premises. Similarly, for adults in the workplace, "if caught smoking, the fine would be Rs 5,000 for the institution, if two persons are caught, it would be Rs 10,000, while if three persons are caught, it would be Rs 15,000," former health minister Anbumani Ramadoss told reporters in New Delhi, 2006. The government is also planning to increase the fine for individuals smoking in public places from Rs 200 to Rs 1,000, he told them. Expressing concern over the increase in the number of smokers in the country, he said the health ministry has recommended the formulation of a comprehensive tobacco control policy and its effective implementation needs to be initiated. "There is a need to increase awareness among teachers, students and community leaders," he said at the release of the *Global Youth Tobacco Survey and Global School Personnel Survey 2006*. Observing that the high prevalence of tobacco use among students and school personnel is alarming, the survey said that indications of increasing tobacco use among girls in some regions is also a matter of concern. Currently, use of tobacco products other than cigarettes by students in the age group of 13–15 years has increased at the national level. According to the survey, six out of ten schools do not follow a tobacco-free policy. While as many as 48.4 per cent schools in North India do not allow smoking within their campuses, the number stands at just 22 per cent in East India. Nearly four out of every five school personnel reported never having received anti-tobacco training to prevent youth from tobacco use. Almost two of every three school personnel reported that their schools did not have non-classroom alcohol control activities. They also said they had no access to teaching materials on tobacco. The findings listed in Tables 10 and 11 throw up the very encouraging fact that after the anti-tobacco training, students were sensitized against tobacco use, motivated to act as monitors for tobacco control, and ready to take part in all tobacco control activities.

Reactions of Teachers

Table 10.13 *Percentage Distribution of Teachers According to the Usefulness of Tobacco Control Activities*

(N = 5)

Activities	*Great Extent (%)*	*Less Extent (%)*
Drawing competition	100	—
Illustrative talk on harmful effects of tobacco	100	—
Expert talk	100	—
Games	100	—
Role Play	100	—
Play	100	—
Yoga	80	20
Movie	100	—
Medical check-ups	100	—
Essay competition	80	20

Table 10.13 indicates that all the teachers – 100 per cent – agreed that the activities under the tobacco control project helped the students to learn about the harmful effects of tobacco consumption. Around 20 per cent of the teachers said they felt that some of the activities, such as Yoga and the essay competition, helped the students only to a certain extent.

Table 10.14 *Percentage Distribution of Teachers According to their Opinion on Whether the Students Enjoyed All the Project Activities*

Teachers' Opinion	*Yes (%)*	*No (%)*
Activities enjoyed by the students	100	—

Table 10.14 indicates that all the teachers – 100 per cent – agreed that the students enjoyed all the activities of the project.

Table 10.15 indicates that all the teachers – 100 per cent – felt that the project worker was able to manage all the activities under the project and keep the students interested. The table also shows that the project worker was able to select the relevant activities for tobacco control education.

Table 10.15 *Percentage Distribution of Teachers Regarding the Project Worker*

Project Worker	*Yes (%)*	*No (%)*
Could manage all the activities properly	100	—
Could select relevant anti-tobacco activities	100	—
Could sustain the interest of the students in tobacco control activities	100	—

Table 10.16 *Percentage Distribution of Teachers Regarding Future Tobacco Control Activities*

Future Recommendations	*Yes (%)*	*No (%)*
Every school should have information on tobacco control	100	—
Activities relating to tobacco control must be given importance in the future	100	—
There any change in students while performing tobacco control activities	100	—

Table 10.16 indicates that all the teachers – 100 per cent – agreed that there should be more such efforts to raise awareness about the harmful effects of tobacco among the students.

Conclusion and Suggestions

The Department of Extension and Communication has been working for community development since the past many years and it has been focusing on the health aspect in particular. Its members are experts in developing and using teaching aids, such as leaflets, posters, films, booklets and flip charts, which are highly effective means of spreading developmental messages. The objective of the anti-tobacco project was to sensitize schoolchildren about the ill effects of tobacco so that they do not indulge in its consumption and also to get them to promote the message to others in their families and community, so that they can help build a healthy community and society. The future of any nation depends on its children, so such efforts, which are dynamic, contextually relevant and need based, will help in shaping all human development.

Bibliography

Bynner, J.M. 1969. *The Young Smoker*. London. Her Majesty's Stationary Office.

Hora, Mahendra and Singh, Kikani N.B. 1991. *A Cytological Study of Sputum in Tobacco Smokers and Non-Smoker in Vadodara*. The MS University of Baroda, Vadodara.

http: //kidshealth.org/teen/drug_alcohol/tobacco/smokeless.html

Mahadevan, K. 1992. *Health Education for Quality of Life*. B.R. Publishing Corp., Delhi.

Ministry of Education Pamphlet No. 31. 2002. 'Health Education: A Hand Book of Suggestions for the Consideration of Teachers and Others Concerned in the Health Education of Children and Young People'. 1956. Reprinted by Her Majesty's Stationary Office, London.

Singh, Uttam Kumar and Nayak, A.K. 1997. *Health Education*. Common Wealth Publishers, New Delhi.

The Times of India, Ahmedabad edition, Friday, 21 March 2008.

The Times of India, Ahmedabad edition, Monday, 19 November 2007.

The Times of India, Ahmedabad edition, Saturday, 27 October 2007.

The Times of India, Ahmedabad edition, Tuesday, 18 January 2008.

The Times of India, Ahmedabad edition, Tuesday, 25 March 2008.

The Times of India, Ahmedabad edition, Friday, 21 March 2008.

www.indiantobacco.com

www.tobaccofreekids.org

www.streetdrugs.org/tobacco.htm

11 Health Clubs

A Healthy Foundation for Tomorrow

One definition of health offered by Anderson and Creswell (1978) states that health is "... that quality of physical, emotional and mental well-being that is enjoyable". Though the terms used to define health may differ, the definitions are generally quite similar in meaning. Most definitions remind us that health has many dimensions, including the physical, mental, emotional, social and even spiritual ones. The fact that the various definitions stress these different dimensions reflects the very personal nature of health. Of course, the dimensions of health are related and each dimension affects the others. Since one's health may change from week to week, month to month and year to year, we can also say that health is not absolute, that it is relative to a particular time or event in life. Anderson and Creswell's definition of health fits well with school health programmes. School health programmes are organized plans of action to promote the well-being of each and every child so that they can live effectively and enjoyably, both in and out of school. This goal is accomplished through the three distinct, but related, components of school health programmes: health services, a healthful school environment and health instruction.

Health Education

The World Health Organization Expert Committee on Health Education of the Public (1954) says: "Health education, like general education, is concerned with changes in the knowledge, feelings and behaviours of people. In its most usual forms, it concentrates on developing such health practices as are believed to bring about the best state possible of well-being." "Health education comprises consciously constructed opportunities for learning, involving some form of communication designed to improve health literacy, including improving knowledge and developing life skills that are conducive to individual and community health." (Singh and Nayak, 1997)

Health education is a 'process', which is carefully planned and effectively conducted with appropriate consideration of the ultimate goals and the best means for reaching them. Although unplanned experiences contribute to an individual's health education, health education is concerned with supplementing incidental experiences with those that are carefully selected for their known values in attaining specific goals. Health education is an abstract term that means different things to different people. To some, it is a matter of public relations aimed at publicizing the activities of health departments and winning public goodwill. Some consider it synonymous with propaganda, that is, the spreading of specific systematized knowledge about health. Many equate it with the transmission of knowledge from expert professionals to lay clients. Health education attempts to close the gap between what is known about optimum health practices and what is actually practised.

Importance of Health Education in Schools

Schools are responsible in many ways for the mental, physical, moral and spiritual development of the future citizens of the country, although the responsibility of the family, government and other concerned persons in this regard can in no way be ignored. Therefore, it is the sacred duty of schools to give a prominent place to health education and direct its schemes in the interest of the growth of children. So far, our schools have failed miserably in this respect, as have our educational authorities. The sooner this state of affairs ends, the better. It is true that India is so poor that most of our children do not get a balanced and nutritious diet, which is why people say that it is a farce to talk of health education for children when they are not even getting proper food to eat. But it is also true that we are deprived of the maximum advantage of even our poor resources because of our ignorance of basic health rules. It is thus necessary to remove this ignorance. The state, school, family and other significant players should all cooperate in planning an active health education programme, which will contribute to the building of a bright future for our children.

Need for Creating Health Clubs in Schools

Childhood is the most joyful period of life. It is a time of immense creative energy, self-discovery and exploration of the world. Children are like growing creepers – they can be moulded as we want. They can also be fraught with feelings of isolation, loneliness and confusion because of various factors in their physical, social, emotional, mental and spiritual well-being. Schools, families and communities need to play a positive and responsible role in bringing up children in a healthful environment that will enable them to maximize their potential. Schools are important for the cognitive, creative and social development of children. They can be dynamic settings for promoting health and for enabling children to grow and mature into healthy adults. Yet, the potential of schools to enhance health is often underutilized. 'School health' has remained confined largely to medical check-ups of children or some hours of health instruction in the curriculum. There is a growing recognition that the physical and psychosocial well-being of children and youth is of fundamental value and schools can provide a strategic means of improving children's health, self-esteem, life skills and behaviour. Although schools have undertaken several initiatives in promoting school health, comprehensiveness and sustainability were not clearly laid out in these initiatives. The need of the hour is a comprehensive school health policy integrated within the school system.

In 2006, the Central Board of Secondary Education (CBSE) suggested that all schools must plan out a 'comprehensive school health programme', which could be initiated through 'health clubs' in each school. Healthy living, especially of schoolchildren, is a prime concern of all stakeholders, including principals, parents, teachers and the community. Collective responsibility has to be assumed to achieve this objective. Important dimensions here are that of experience and development of health skills and physique through practical engagements, such as play, exercise, sports and practice of personal and community hygiene. Health and wellness clubs in schools will focus on children's overall well-being, comprising their emotional, social and mental health. They will act as enabling and organizational points for conducting activities related to the various dimensions of health and wellness. Such institutions will offer the school's students health cards, which will serve as links for their growth and development. The health cards will also form an effective monitoring and feedback system for the overall health of children while at school. Thus, a project was started to set up an experimental health club in a school in Vadodara city, the T.R. Patel School in Sardar Nagar, with the following specific objectives:

- To develop understanding amongst the school's students regarding the concept, structure and functions of health clubs.
- To teach the students Yoga and meditation techniques from an early age.
- To motivate them to adopt good hygienic practices.
- To make them conscious of good, healthy eating habits.
- To organize health based activities that would improve their health status through the health club.

Methodology

The very first step of the project was to plan the intended course of action. Systematic planning provides guidelines to implement a project successfully. The plan of action includes the list of activities to be conducted for a particular period of time. It answers major questions about the project, such as where, when, how and by whom. In this project, the content for the activities of the health club was selected after consulting the list of activities laid out by the CBSE and by referring to books on health education. The project worker also referred to a report on health fairs, compiled by Chetana, a child resource centre based in Ahmedabad. Thus, it was finally decided that the health club would offer knowledge and activities on:

- Yoga
- Medical check-ups

- Mental health
- Sanitation
- Nutrition
- Recreation

Contacting Resource People

The project worker contacted resource people and asked them to help her start the health club with their advice and suggestions on how to conduct activities such as medical check-ups and expert talks.

Table 11.1 *Experts Invited for Conducting Health Education Sessions*

Topic	*Resource Person*
Medical Check-Ups	Dr Navin Patel (physician)
Expert Talk on Mental Health	Dr Kritaghna Singh (psychologist)
Yoga	Ms Bhagyasheela Panchal (yoga expert)
Meditation	Ms Bhagyasheela Panchal (meditation instructor)

Preparing Teaching Aids

Teaching aids help learners understand a concept easily. Several experiments have shown that teaching aids can help make a programme successful. Teaching aids were both prepared and borrowed for use in the activities of the health club.

Table 11.2 *Different Types of Teaching Aids Used in the Project*

Teaching Aids	*Topics*
Posters	Importance of nutritive food – illustrative talk
	Yoga – illustrative talk
	Introduction of the health club
Flip Charts	Importance of nutritious – illustrative talk
	Yoga – illustrative talk
Flash Cards	Summarizing the points of dustbin making
Placards	Messages on hygienic practices – Snakes and Ladders game

Selection of the Target Group

First the school was identified. Then the venue, timings and members of the health club were decided, after which the students were contacted.

Identifying the School

The project worker contacted two schools in Vadodara initially, Nutan Vidhyalay on New Sama Road and T.R. Patel School in Sardar Nagar. The principals of these schools were given an orientation in the concept of health clubs. The principal of Nutan Vidhyalay said they were not interested because they followed hectic academic schedules. But after several discussions and meetings, the principal of T.R. Patel School was convinced about the need to start a health club in his school.

Deciding the Venue, Time and Health Club Members

A meeting was held with the administrative staff and the principal of the school to decide the venue and timing for the health club activities. The administrative staff and the principal of the school allotted three days each – Monday, Tuesday and Wednesday – from 7.30 am to 9.30 am for the health club activities. The venue for the activities was the school's assembly hall.

Contacting the Students

The students of Class 6 were contacted for membership of the health club because it was felt that their age was appropriate to understanding health concepts. Their interest in health activities was assessed and then they were given an orientation about the health club, which was to be established in the school with their help.

Table 11.3 *Schedule of Health Club Activities*

Activity	*Content*
Orientation	About the health club
Motivational Games	Recreational
Medical Check-Ups	Height, weight and cleanliness of nails, ears, tongue, hands, etc.

Poster Making	Slogans on health and hygiene
Discussion	'Health is Wealth'
Crossword Game	Nutritious food
Demonstration	Dustbin making
Workshop	Best out of the West
Cleanliness Drive	Cleanliness of the school
Yoga	Practising yoga, its advantages and its rules and regulations
Meditation	Mental concentration
Snakes and Ladders Game	Hygienic practices
Demonstration	First aid box
Expert Talk	Mental well-being
Puppet Show	Nutritive value of vegetables and fruits
Play	'Health is Wealth'
Orientation for Teachers	Yoga, mental heath, plastic bags, how they can impart health education to students while teaching other courses
Valedictory Function	Displays of material prepared by health club members and teaching aids used in health club activities

Inauguration of the Project

The inauguration and orientation of the project were conducted by the members of the health club, who were the principal, Mr Vadi Bhai Shah, the Class VIth teacher, Ms Dhanlaxmi Ben Pandit, and 45 boys and girls of Class VIth.

There should be an excellent rapport between the members and the project worker if the project is to be effective. Different motivational games were played and a story telling session was organized to build a rapport among the members of the health club and the project worker. The health club was inaugurated on 13 November 2006.

Activities Conducted under the Health Club

Here are the details of the activities conducted by the health club in T.R. School, Vadodara:

Orientation

Objective: To orient the students about the health club and its activities.

Activity: With the help of a teacher coordinator, the project worker explained to the students the concept of a health club and told them about the kind of activities that took place there. The teacher coordinator talked about health and the importance of health care. The project worker convinced the students to join the health club.

Motivational Activity

Objective: To built a rapport with the members of the health club.

Activity: The club members were made to stand in a circle. One of them would say 'big ball' while enacting that he/she was holding a small ball. The next student in the circle would say 'small ball' and enact holding a big ball. Any student who spoke or enacted wrong had to move out of the game. This game helped to dispel any shyness in the group members and also to build a rapport between them.

Medical Check-Ups

Objective: To check the height, weight and cleanliness of the members of the health club.

Activity: The project worker invited a doctor to conduct medical check-ups of the members of the health club. Dr Navin Patel checked their height, weight and the state of their eyes, hair, ears, tongue, hands and nails. Dr Patel also gave them health tips, such as washing their hands when they came in from play, before eating and after using the toilet, and not sitting too close to the television while watching a programme. He also suggested they undergo regular medical check-ups to keep an eye on their health status.

Gain: The students became aware of their health status and they became conscious of the need to take care of their eyes, hands, nails, hair, ears, etc.

Poster Making Competition

Objective: To help the students understand the importance of cleanliness for good health.

Activity: The club members were divided into 15 groups, with three members in each group, and given a slogan related to cleanliness. They were given chart paper and colouring materials and asked to make a poster. The project worker instructed them in how to write slogans, draw pictures and colour them. They were given three hours to finish their posters. Three winners were announced and given motivational gifts. The competition was followed by a discussion on the topic of the competition, 'Health is Wealth'.

Gain: The students became aware of the importance of health and cleanliness for good health. They learnt to coordinate and work in a group and were able to develop their ability to discuss health issues.

Crossword Game

Objective: To make the students aware of the various kinds of nutritive foods in their daily food intake.

Activity: The project worker wrote the name of one nutritive food on the blackboard, then a student had to come forward and write another name from the nutritive food group, matching the last letter in the first name, much in the same fashion as Antakshari, the song game, is played.

Gain: The students became aware of the various kinds of nutritive food and their value in their daily lives.

Dustbin Making

Objective: To help the students make dustbins.

Activity: The project worker showed the club members how to make a dustbin. Then, the members were divided into 15 groups, each of which made a dustbin out of waste cardboard boxes, coloured paper and colours. The students wrote attractive messages on the dustbins and drew pictures and cartoons on them.

Gain: The students were able to develop their creative skills and make something useful in maintaining cleanliness – a dustbin.

Cleanliness Drive

Objective: To promote cleanliness in the school campus.

Activity: The students used the dustbins they had prepared earlier in this activity. They had to clean the school campus. The project worker gave them instructions and divided them into nine groups, allocating a specific area of the school to each group.

Gain: The students learnt that they have to put in an effort to keep their school clean.

Yoga

Objective: To teach the students Yoga techniques.

Activity: A Yoga expert, Ms Bhagyasheela Panchal, was invited to teach the club members the techniques of Yoga. At the end of the session, the project worker gave an illustrative talk on the advantages and rules and regulations of Yoga with the help of flip charts and charts.

Gain: The students learnt the techniques of Yoga and were made aware of its advantages and limitations.

Meditation

Objective: To teach the students meditation techniques.

Activity: Ms Panchal, who is also a teacher of meditation, was invited to teach the students meditation techniques. At the end of the session, the project worker discussed the advantages and rules and regulations of meditation. For the purposes of evaluation, the project worker asked members to come forward and write on the blackboard the advantages of meditation; each point was then discussed by the group.

Gain: The students learnt meditation techniques as also their advantages, rules and regulations.

Snakes and Ladders Game

Objective: To motivate the students to adopt hygienic practices.

Activity: The project worker brought the game from the Department of Extension and Communication, Faculty of Family and Community Sciences, MS University of Baroda, Vadodara. She prepared flash cards with messages to put on the Snakes and Ladders game sheet. The game sheet was spread on the floor and the flash cards of correct and wrong hygienic practices placed at the bottom of the ladders and at the mouths of the snakes, respectively. The project worker then gave instructions on how to play the game and its rules and regulations. Five students began the game; whenever any of the playing members won or got out of the game, new members were added.

Gain: The students realized that if they follow good hygienic practices in their lives, they will enjoy good health and live longer.

Demonstration

Objective: Tou make the students aware of a first aid box and its use.

Activity: The project worker demonstrated how to prepare a first aid box and what it should contain. She also gave an illustrative talk on the use of the first aid box.

Gain: The students became aware of the uses of a first aid box.

Expert Talk: Mental Well-Being

Objective: To orient the students about mental health and its importance in our lives.

Activity: Dr Kritaghna Singh, a psychologist, was invited to give a talk on mental well-being. He talked about the concept of mental health and the importance of mental well-being in our lives. Dr Singh also talked to the students about the disadvantages of anger and its deleterious effects on our minds.

Gain: The students became aware about the importance of mental well-being and the bad effects of anger on the human mind.

Puppet Show

Objective: To make the students aware of the nutritive values of fruit and vegetables.

Activity: During the puppet show, short jingles were sung about the nutritive value of fruits and vegetables. At the end, with the help of a puppet character, the students were asked questions such as: What nutrient does a banana contain? (Calcium) What are carrots good for? (Eyes).

Gain: The students became aware of the nutritive values of fruits and vegetables. They also became aware of how nutrition can help our bodies grow.

Play

Objective: To explain to the students the importance of cleanliness for good health.

Activity: A play on the topic, 'Health is Wealth', was prepared by ten students. Ready scripts were given to them and, after several rehearsals, they were ready to perform for the health club. The play's theme was the importance of cleanliness for good health. After the play was performed, the project worker discussed the messages sent out by the play.

Gain: The students were made aware of the direct relationship between cleanliness and good health.

Orientation Programme for Teachers

An orientation programme for the teachers of T.R. Patel School was organized on 8 February 2007at the health club. Twelve of the 15 teachers in the school participated in the orientation programme. The programme focused on inculcating health skills through school activities, while dealing with various other subjects. The project worker oriented the teachers in Yoga and mental health. She also showed the teachers different ways to disseminate health information through various school activities and subjects, as, for example, a sports competition celebrating Cleanliness Day, medical check-ups, Yoga classes and the maintenance of a clean and healthy environment.

Valedictory Function

The health club project was completed in two months, at the end of which a valedictory function was arranged in the school.

Findings

An evaluation of the project revealed that all the members of the health club – 100 per cent – found the Snakes and Ladders game, crossword game, poster competition and Yoga session most interesting. A very large majority of them – 97.78 per cent – found the meditation and dustbin making activities very interesting. A majority of the members found the play, puppet show, cleaning drive, discussion and illustrative talk interesting. A few of the members said they did not find the medical check-ups very interesting.

This shows that all of the members found the games the most effective. A very large majority of the members – 97.78 per cent – found the play, puppet show and poster competition more effective. A few of the members – 6.67 per cent – found the medical check-ups and expert talk less effective. All the members felt that Yoga could help to maintain physical fitness to a great extent. A large majority of the members – 95.56 per cent – felt that meditation helped to maintain concentration and that the cleaning drive helped to promote cleanliness in the school to a great extent. Around 15.56 per cent of the members said that dustbins could help in controlling garbage.

The evaluation revealed that a very large majority of the members – 95.56 per cent – started washing their hands more often and eating all the food put before them. A large majority of the members – 91.11 per cent – started washing their hands before eating and practising meditation and avoiding anger; 26.67 per cent said they had begun practising Yoga. All the members – 100 per cent – said more games, competitions and Yoga classes should be arranged under the health club, whereas a large majority of the members suggested that regular medical check-ups should be conducted.

When the teachers of the school were asked about the project, all of them – 100 per cent – agreed that the health club activities had helped the students to learn about health. Around 20 per cent of the teachers said that some of the activities, such as Yoga, meditation and the Snakes and Ladders game, could not help the students to learn about health. All the teachers – 100 per cent – said they needed support to organize future health related activities. Around 60 per cent of the teachers said they needed support to invite experts. All of them said they needed support to get more money to run the health club.

Follow-up

After the completion of the project, a follow-up was done to check on the status of the health club that was planned and initiated at the T.R. Patel School with the help of its teachers and the students. The results were found to be encouraging and motivating. Mr Vadi Bhai Shah, the principal of the school, had given the health club a corner and some storage space as he had promised. All the teaching materials, such as the charts, flash cards, puppets and Yoga booklet, which had been prepared and used by the project worker, were kept properly and used by the club members under the supervision of their class teacher, who was very actively involved in the project. It was observed that the children in the school were more alert and sensitive towards clean classrooms, a clean school building and a clean environment; for example, they were using the dustbins they had made during the project. These observations were very encouraging as improving the sanitation and cleanliness of schools and the development of life skills are an essential investment both in the short and long term for future generations of schoolchildren and their families.

Conclusion

On the basis of the above observations and findings, one can conclude that health clubs are an effective way of imparting health education to schoolchildren. Effective teaching methods, such as games, plays, puppet shows, discussions, competitions and exercise sessions, can be used with a participatory approach involving both teachers and students. Non-governmental organizations and voluntary organizations can also collaborate with schools by providing the teaching materials or facilities to run health clubs.

Bibliography

Chaube, S.P. 1964. *Health Education: A Text Book for Pupil-Teachers*. Kailash Printing Press, Agra.

Engs, Ruth and Wantz, Molly. 1978. *Teaching Health Education in Elementary Schools*. Houghton Mifflin Co., Boston.

Mahadevan, K. 1992. *Health Education for Quality of Life*. B.R. Publishing Corp., Delhi.

Ministry of Education Pamphlet No. 31. 'Health Education: A Hand Book of Suggestions for the Consideration of Teachers and Others Concerned in the Health and Education of Children and Young People'. 1956. Reprinted by Her Majesty's Stationary Office, London.

Modi, Rachana. 2005. 'An Action Project on Starting a Value Education Centre in a School of Baroda City'. MSc project. Department of Extension and Communication, Faculty of Home Science, MS University of Baroda, Vadodara.

Rana, Ansuya. 1971. 'Knowledge and Practice regarding Personal Health and Sanitation of the Eight Standard Students of Village Asoj'. MSc project. Department of Extension and Communication, Faculty of Home Science, MS University of Baroda, Vadodara.

Seth, Divya. 2003. 'An Action Project to Start an Eco-Club in a Higher Secondary School of Baroda City'. MSc project. Department of Extension and Communication, Faculty of Home Science, MS University of Baroda, Vadodara

Singh, Uttam Kumar and Nayak, A.K. 1997. *Health Education*. Commonwealth Publishers, New Delhi.

Webliography

wordnet.princeton.edu
www.apllohospdelhi.com
www.cbse.nic.in
www.dph.state.ct.us
www.miea.or.jp
www.mypurohith.com/yoga
www.sanicom.net
nutritionfoundationofindia.res.in

12 Importance of Recreation in the Life of Women

The word 'recreation' originates from the Latin word, 'recreatio', meaning to restore or refresh. Recreation is the feeling of well-being that results from experiences in which people receive a pleasurable and gratifying response to the use of their physical, mental or creative powers. It is the essence of any experience through which people directly gain personal enjoyment and satisfaction. It is a distinct phase of human activity, characterized by a particular spirit or attitude, which brings about direct satisfaction of human needs. Recreational activities are relaxing to human beings and provide diversions from their normal routine. They are a kind of refreshment of the mind and the body. They are more like tools and, because they are in tune with nature, they are an essential part of living and of direct benefit to individuals. To have value as recreation, activities must be suited to one's physical, mental and emotional needs. Recreation is viewed as any activity or pursuit that is chosen voluntarily by the participants within their leisure time, with the primary motivation of achieving personal pleasure and with a minimum of other hoped for goals or compulsions surrounding it.

Gray M. (1986) defined recreation as "an emotional condition within an individual human being that flows from a feeling of well-being and self-satisfaction. It is characterized by feelings of mastery, achievement, exhilaration, acceptance, success, personal worth and pleasure. It reinforces a positive self-image. Recreation is a response to an aesthetic experience, achievement of personal goals, or positive feedback from others. It is independent of activity, leisure or social acceptance." Recreation is the use of time in a non-profitable way, in many ways also the therapeutic refreshment of one's body or mind. The National Therapeutic Recreation Society (NTRS), Windsor (Canada) defines therapeutic recreation as: "Practised in clinical, residential and community settings, the profession of Therapeutic Recreation uses treatment, education and recreation services to help people with illnesses, disabilities and other conditions to develop and use their leisure in ways that enhance their health, independence and well-being."

Recreation is not a tangible, static thing, but a vital force influencing the lives of people. It is essential to happiness and satisfaction in living. Through recreation, people grow and develop their powers and personality.

Criteria for a Community Recreation Programme

The following may be considered essential criteria for an adequate recreational programme, regardless of the size or type of community or the agency providing it. These criteria are based upon the principle that all such programmes should fulfil individual and social needs, afford outlets for creative expression, and contribute to a fuller life for all the people in the community. They take into account the activities that everyone needs and that have a universal appeal, as well as individual differences and tastes. Every community recreation programme should:

- Provide equal opportunity for both sexes and all ages, not forgetting the sick and the handicapped.
- Include a wide spectrum of activities serving the interests and needs of the people.
- Take into account the widely differing tastes and interests of individuals.
- Offer activities affording varying and progressive degrees of skill and ability.
- Carry over into adult life the skills and interests acquired in school and college.
- Encourage individuals and groups to expand their interests and provide their own activities.

- Involve the active participation of individuals and community groups in planning the programme.
- Utilize fully and wisely all available community resources, both human and physical.
- Provide recreational opportunities within the financial abilities of all the community members.
- Undergo continuous constructive evaluation.

Recreation plays a vital role in a community:

- When significant physical, creative, emotional, social and creative outcomes are derived from recreation for each individual, it enhances the quality of living in the community as a whole.
- When children, youth, adult men, women and older citizens are all engaged in challenging and stimulating forms of leisure activity, or in helping to plan and organize community or agency programmes of recreation, this inevitably aids in creating a community in which desirable social values are stressed.
- When individuals learn habits and attitudes of group cooperation and responsibility, they are inevitably better able to conduct themselves as effective citizens within the structure of neighbourhood and community life.
- Many of the problems that plague our modern society may be ameliorated by the imaginative provision of recreational services, facilities and personnel.
- Provision of adequate recreational experiences will help women to emerge from boredom, apathy, and physical and psychological degeneration. Concerted efforts should be made to solve this problem, through the development and support of recreational programmes specifically geared to meet the needs of women.

Principles of Recreation

- Each individual needs to discover which activities give him/her personal satisfaction. They should be helped to develop the essential skills in these.

- Each individual should be helped to form a habit of finding pleasure in reading.
- Each individual should be encouraged to discover one or more hobbies.
- Ultimate satisfaction in recreation comes only through one's own achievement – of whatever kind.

Purposes of Recreational Activities

- To promote and enhance the quality of life.
- To offer activities that are meaningful to each individual.
- To enhance or maintain cognitive abilities.
- To enhance or maintain physical abilities.
- To promote emotional and psychosocial well-being.
- To provide opportunities for socialization.
- To offer opportunities for creative expression.
- To offer opportunities for decision making, choice and responsibility.
- To offer opportunities for religious or spiritual expression.
- To offer solace and relaxation.
- To provide opportunities for fun, pleasure and enjoyment.
- To offer opportunities to share common interests, cultures and experiences.
- To provide opportunities to learn new skills, adapt old skills, and enjoy new leisure experiences.

Characteristics of Recreation

- What one person views as recreational activity may not be so for another. Indeed, an activity may be recreational for an individual at a given time and place, and not in another.
- People engage in recreational activity because they desire and choose to do so, without compulsion of any type other than an urge from within. It is not a forced activity.
- People find opportunities for self-expression in recreational activities and derive fun, relaxation and pleasure from them.
- It represents a medium through which the personality achieves satisfying expression and which contributes to human happiness.

- It may be socially constructive and serve important personal and social needs, or it may represent degrading, time-wasting or even antisocial or criminal forms of activity.

Importance of Recreational Activities

In the days gone by, recreation was seen as a reward for work well done, and it was intended to prepare people for more work. Today, of course, as work has become less laborious and demanding, this traditional view of the function of recreation has become less widely accepted. It is no longer necessary to see it in relation to economically productive activity; it is productive and valuable in its own right.

Personal Values of Recreational Experience

Probably the most important single reason why people take part in a recreational experience is that it brings a direct measure of happiness to them. Briefly stated, the direct outcomes of a successful recreational experience for the individual may be listed under the following headings:

Social Outcomes

The social outcomes and values of recreational experience are important for people of all ages, but particularly so for young people. For adolescents and adults as well, a wide variety of satisfying group contacts, in which the individual relates effectively to others, shares their concerns and needs, and is accepted by them as a human being, is essential to social growth.

Creative Outcomes

Recreation permits people to be themselves and to explore their individual, special creative talents. This is particularly true within the aesthetic areas of art, music, theatre, dance and creative writing. In each of these, people are given the opportunity to make a unique expressive statement that is theirs alone. Within recreation, there need not be any limit, and people can be free to fully explore their latent creative abilities.

Physical Outcomes

Recreational activities make an important contribution to the total well-being of people. Participating in sports, games, dance or outdoor activities suited to one's age and general level of health and fitness is one of the surest ways to maintain an effectively functioning cardio-vascular system and good muscular tone.

Emotional Outcomes

The ability to develop hobbies, interests and group ties, to find emotional release through active sports or expressive arts, to find peace and relaxation in a natural setting – all these are part of a well balanced living regimen.

Intellectual Outcomes

Recreation may easily include attending legitimate theatre shows or concerts, a great variety of reading, scientific pursuits, hobbies, exploration and travel, participating in adult courses and seminars, or similar pursuits. Provided that these are not work related and have no other major extrinsic purpose, they are recreationally motivated.

Social Values of Recreation

From a societal point of view, when each member of a community derives significant physical, creative, emotional, social and creative outcomes, it enhances the quality of living in the community as a whole. When children, youth, adults, women and older citizens are all engaged in challenging, stimulating forms of leisure activity, or in helping to plan and organize community or agency programmes of recreation, this inevitably aids in creating a community in which desirable social values are stressed.

Economic Values of Recreation

In an economic sense, the importance of leisure and recreation for the nation is tremendous. It comprises a major industry and absorbs a considerable portion of our productive energies.

Each year, large new markets and fields of employment are being developed. What is not always so clearly understood is the extent to which recreation has positive economic value for the communities in which it exists. For every community, the extent to which it has come to grips with its recreational needs may prove an important asset or serious liability. Nothing is more important to the physical and emotional health of men and women.

Recreational Needs and Women

Women's mental health issues are gaining ground in the women's studies discourse. The women's movement has provided fresh inputs in terms of individual and group counselling, popularly known as 'consciousness raising' exercises, a form of mutual counselling that enables women as a group to share their experiences, problems, feelings, dreams and action plans for rebuilding shattered lives. This process of attaining feminist consciousness allows women to recognize that what they perceive as personal problems can be shared with others in a non-threatening and non-power oriented atmosphere. It also enables women to realize what they think of as a result of living in a patriarchal society. It empowers women to come to a realization of their own potential and makes them autonomous, self-dependent in their decision making, and emotionally self-reliant. It is an ongoing process that brings about personal and collaborative change as opposed to structural change. The need for small groups and informal group discussions is emphasized in this method.

Manifestations of Depression

Depression manifests in women as headaches, insomnia, constant tension, detachment, irritability, loss of appetite, dryness of the mouth, fear, self-blame, lack of concentration and lack of interest in any kind of activity. Although chronic headaches may not be psychosomatic, they can also be caused by depression or anxiety. Counselling can help to identify and address emotional concerns and should be considered as part of the treatment.

Two types of stress lead to mental disorders. The biochemical stressors are hormonal fluctuations at the onset of puberty, in the premenstrual phase, in the post-partum phase and during menopause. An imbalance in serotonin levels has, in fact, been implicated in disorders such as migraine and depression. Psychosocial stressors originate from the external social environment, such as women's inferior social position, lack of power, homelessness, economic hardships, and manmade or natural disasters. They create helplessness (women's seeming passivity in the midst of crises such as domestic violence, accidents, etc.) and reduce the motivation to lead an active life. Stress related mental health issues are also caused by illness in the family, the death of one's spouse, divorce or an accident that might reduce or destroy a woman's ability to shoulder responsibility. Women get displaced after marriage, which brings about cultural loss and bereavement, loss of social networks and support systems, and loss of traditional healing sites. The psychological stages through which women pass are enduring, suffering, reckoning, reconciling and normalizing. The successful completion of this therapeutic cycle depends on how conducive their physical and emotional systems are. Women cope with tension by crying, talking it over, praying, and engaging in creative work such as music, art, craft, reading, studies, community work and team building.

In India, the focus is more on the treatment of an ailment, seldom on preventive and promotive efforts. Marginalization of mental health concerns results from the understanding that mental distress is a manifestation of an individual problem, not directly related to social oppression and not common to all women.

Another different approach emphasizes cross-cultural psychiatry and evaluates the phenomenon of mental illness from within a culture. Traditional treatments for mental ailments used to be meditation, Yoga, group singing and listening to religious discourses. Culturally sensitive counselling on mental health and the consequences of trauma takes into consideration women's sociocultural environment. The two approaches have given way to a new cross-cultural psychiatry where the emphasis is on the different contexts of mental illness in different cultures, not on biomedical categories. Now, there are no two opinions about the statement that psychotherapy should take into consideration the multicultural aspects of women's existential reality.

The four phases of the therapeutic or healing cycle are:

- *Enduring:* anxiety, grieving and loss of partner.
- *Acceptance:* reality testing, preparedness and reckoning of the future, reconciling, evaluation of self and resources, recuperating.
- *Recovery:* rebuilding life, maximizing options, setting new goals, healing
- *Normalizing:* stability and routines, building relationships and community.

An unequal relationship between the professional counsellor, who is 'up there', and the patient, who is 'down below', creates a communication gap. In the case of women, this inequality is compounded by their subjugation under the patriarchal psychiatric system.

Experiences from both industrialized and developing countries have revealed that the prevalence of common mental disorders or minor psychiatric morbidity is high among the urban low income and marginalized population. The women in these segments are even more vulnerable. Globalization, the Structural Adjustment Programmes, increasing conflict with neighbouring countries, and the ongoing sectarian violence in the country along caste, ethnic and communal lines have put Indian women at high risk of mental illness.

Recreational Activities for Women

Media

People engage in television viewing because there is a vacuum in their lives. Different standards of morality for men and women are present in the messages sent out by films, television serials and advertisements. Adolescent girls working as domestic workers don't have any emotional support because there are hardly any television and radio programmes for them. Magazines and newspapers can help women to entertain themselves. Women can be helped by the promotion of women's agency in the media so that they can lead intellectually, psychologically and emotionally self-sufficient lives.

Counselling in Women's Shelters

The most promising solution to confusion and disorientation among the inmates of women's shelters is a democratic space for brainstorming because autism of anxiety is one of the main problems faced by them. An informal set-up is more congenial for their personal and career counselling. Workers at women's shelters need to understand that there is a story behind every kind of behaviour. It is important for them to know that story. A panel of psychotherapists and psychoanalysts should conduct staff development programmes at women's shelters so that the staff can handle post-trauma stress disorders among the inmates with empathy, instead of resorting to blame tactics. Recreational activities can prove to be of great use in women's shelters.

Role of Support and Self-Help Groups (SHGs)

Self-help groups (SHGs) provide a democratic space for rebuilding broken lives. Non-power oriented special interest groups provide stimuli for the channelling of creative energy. Mutual counselling and focusing on experience sharing without preaching can help psychologically distressed women reorganize their lives and enhance their potential. 'Speak out centres' can provide a platform for community mental health intervention. Here comes the endorsement from well-known expert of gender studies, Prof. Amita Verma, "At the height of feminist activism in the 1970s and 1980s, there was excitement in the air as women shared experiences about themselves, their families, their lives and encounters." The growth of women's confidence and self-esteem knew no bounds as they challenged the established theories on law, work, justice, equality and medicine. They talked late into the night, wrote pamphlets, stuck posters on walls, spoke at public meetings and filed writ petitions. They felt reassured that theirs was not an isolated or individual problem. The group's endorsement and sharing of painful experiences perhaps did much more for mental health than all the medicines in the pharmacopeia. The women's movement helped avert many mental breakdowns. Enduring therapeutic engagement at the community level can include group singing, festival celebrations, discourses on women's issues and public meetings, which help them relax and are also a means of recreation.

Training Programmes in Counselling

Sensitization and training of general practitioners and other health personnel in mental health problems, particularly minor psychiatric morbidity (anxiety and/or depression), are a must. At health posts and public hospitals, there is a need for social counsellors who are in touch with non-governmental organizations (NGOs) that provide institutional support to women in social distress. The sensitization of teachers, community workers, and people who work with youth groups and women's organizations is extremely important. Training sessions for professional and para-professional volunteers should focus on supportive networks, group cohesion and solidarity. Training should include modules on interviewing skills, history taking and mental status examination. The electronic and print media should be trained in sensitizing the general public about the psychological response to violence and providing information about referral services because women and children affected by domestic violence and manmade or social disasters have special psychological needs.

Despite the abject poverty, hard work and everyday struggles involved in a subsistence oriented lifestyle, women have their own ways of enjoying their leisure time. They have an amazing capacity to turn some of their routine work into avenues of recreation and thereby transform some of their driest work into a rewarding leisure experience. Women handle the whole family. They support their children, husbands, fathers and brothers. They provide both mental and moral support to their families. Men have a number of social options, such as reading the newspaper, hanging out with friends, and going to the club. Activities that women can undertake are:

- Cooking classes
- Jewellery making
- Dancing and singing
- Discussions with friends
- Indoor sports such as board games
- Walking and going to the gym

- Reading the newspaper
- Going out with friends

The socialization process of girls and women has fostered the belief that women are less capable, less physically skilled, and poorer in decision making than men. But this sociolizing practices may be one of the best ways to begin to counter this view. Often, the benefits may be recognized in retrospect as the women acknowledge the strengths, skills and self-esteem that they have gained. Women will involve themselves in recreational activities because they give them a break from their routine activities. A constraint to women's involvement may have to do with the way in which they conform to gender expectations. We cannot deny that women's roles in society have changed, but a sense that gender expectations are important still remains. For example, some women may not participate in certain activities because of their perceived gender inappropriateness. In other cases, the roles expected of women will result in their being directed into particular roles because they are confined to traditional roles. The major aspects of the ethic of care relate to responsibility and commitment to others. Most women are socialized into an ethic of care. Thus, they may be constrained in their own personal leisure and in participating in outdoor activities if they are continually putting the needs of others ahead of their own needs. Even within certain activities, the experience may be less satisfying because of the requirements of the ethic of care. For example, women have described how going on a camping trip with their family is not leisure if they have to do all the packing and food preparation and are responsible for making sure that everyone else enjoys the trip.

Women are always busy with their work. Working women have to complete their office work and their household work. Recreation gives them some refreshment from daily work and recharges their abilities and involvement. Recreation helps women to:

- Develop positive attitudes towards life.
- Balance their physical and mental health.
- Build positive self-esteem in terms of increased self-respect and self-integrity.
- Develop and build their creative abilities in different areas.

- Reduce the stress from routine activities.
- We can offer a variety of formats for activities for women only, for mixed groups, and family groups. The varied skill levels of women should be addressed in terms of beginning classes as well as more advanced classes. The amount of structure desired may also vary as some women only need opportunities, while others need instruction and leadership.
- Female leadership can often encourage women who may feel inappropriate in their interests or in their abilities. Women often provide excellent role models to other women so that they can also involve themselves. When women see other women who are skilled and comfortable in the activities, they are more likely to feel that they, too, can perform them.

Recreation Contributes to Happiness

Happiness is essentially a by-product, which can be best achieved through a balanced life. Recreation holds an important place in a balanced life, along with work, rest, love and worship. Life would be incomplete and drab without it. Among the needs for real living are knowledge and ideals, books, pictures, music, songs, dance and games, travel, adventure, romance, friends, companionship and the exchange of minds. Recreation holds its place of importance in modern life because it affords opportunities for the attainment of these basic human needs. The pursuit of happiness, the love of adventure and the desire for achievement are motivating forces which, for large numbers of people, are realized most fully in recreation.

Recreational facilities should always be provided in a culturally sensitive manner and organizers should ensure that girls have equal access to them. The right to 'participate freely in cultural life and the arts' refers to the right to access developmentally appropriate artistic and community events. The quality of play and recreation is directly related to the environment in which they take place.

Conclusion

Recreation is an important aspect of people's lives. Stresses and pressures will keep increasing daily. There has to be some alternative to combat these stresses and keep society healthy, physically, mentally and emotionally. Recreation can help in decreasing stress. Men enjoy their recreational activities on a regular basis, but children, women and elderly people are vulnerable groups that don't get an opportunity for recreation. Thus, emphasis should be put on creating innovative recreational opportunities for women. Women constitute an integral part of society. They play multiple roles and assume multiple responsibilities. Consequently, they face more stress and also need more recreation. Women are seldom involved in attending parties, roaming around and talking on the telephone because they consider these a waste of time and do not value them as recreational activities. Recreational activities are important for ensuring that women remain active and healthy.

Recreation should include activities that women liked to do when they were children and which they are no longer able to do. These activities could include games, music, singing, dancing, cooking classes, art and craft. Some of these can be taken up as hobbies. As we know, recreation is not a tangible, static thing, but a vital force that influences the lives of people. It is essential to happiness and satisfaction in living. Through recreation, people grow and develop their power and personalities. Therefore, it is a matter of public concern that recreation opportunities be made available to everyone.

Bibliography

Alan, J. 2004. *Outdoor Recreation Management*. W.B. Saunders Co., Nothinghum, England.

Butler, G. 1982. *Introduction to Community Recreation*. McGraw Hill Co., London.

Curtis, H. 1987. *Recreation for Teachers*. The Macmillan Co., London.

Kraus, C. 1982. *Creative Management in Recreation Parks and Leisure Services*. Times Mirror College Publishing, London.

Kraus, R. 1984. *Recreation and Leisure in Modern Society*. Printed in North America, Toranto.

Peter, T. and Gratton, C. 2002. *Sports and Recreation: An Analysis*. E & F.N. Spoon Publications, Canada.

Roberson, N. 1986. *Community Health*. Times Mirror College Publishing, London.

Webliography

http: //ace.acadiau.ca/fps/srnik/markham/biblio.htm

http://Lifestyle.indianetzone.com/recreation/1/indoorrecreational activities.htm

http://web1.userinstinct.com/14120364-parks-recreation-elderly recreation-services-punakau-districts-keaau-learning-center.htm

http://www.dirjournal.com/recreation/

http://www.dmoz.org/Recreation/Outdoors/Schooland Education/

http: //www.google.com/Top/Recreation/

http: //www.re-creation.com.au

13 Elderly People and their Recreational Needs

Ageing is a fact of life, and as age advances, people become prone to all types of health disorders. However, if remedial measures are taken at the appropriate time, they can lead active lives till they die. In India, improved health and longevity have changed the definition of what it means to be elderly. Arguably, India's single most stunning achievement during the last century is longevity. In France, it took 120 years for the population of elderly people to double, whereas in India, it has taken just 25 years. The population of elderly people in India has shot up from 12 million in 1901 to 19 million in 1951, 77 million in 2001, and is expected to reach 137 million by 2021.

India now has the second largest ageing population in the world. The UN defines a country as 'ageing' when the proportion of people aged more than 60 years reaches 7 per cent. India has already exceeded this and will reach 12.6 per cent by 2025. But this fast rise in its ageing population adds to India's socioeconomic challenges. Notwithstanding the saying, 'Old is Gold', life for many older people in the country is less than happy. When young people leave their villages for towns and cities, the old are left to fend for themselves. In urban areas, women work outside their homes and, as a result, cease to be the traditional caretakers of old people that they were. Families are becoming more and more nuclear. Their function as a social safety net for elderly people is eroding fast.

Being economically unproductive, elderly people do not have the authority and prestige they enjoyed before and are often perceived as a burden. In industrialized countries, pension systems cover the economic needs of elderly people. In India, where 90 per cent of the total workforce is employed in the informal sector, social security through pension schemes is available to only the 10 per cent who retire from the organized sector. However, the government does offer a pension scheme to destitute people above the age of 65 years. According to a study by Help Age International, only one of every five of those who are eligible under the scheme receives its benefits. Being illiterate and poor, many are not able to even fill in the relevant forms or produce age certificates.

Ageing is a process that begins with conception and continues through life. It is an unavoidable, natural process. As age progresses, there is regression of physical and physiological functions.

Increase in longevity or life span is followed by an increase in the proportion of elderly people in the total population. The year, 1999, was declared the International Year of Older Persons, which was crucial for a country like India, which is going through a revolution in its demographic, economic, social, cultural and psychological status. The ageing of a population is an inevitable consequence of the process of demographic transition and creates an imbalance in the age structure over a period of time. In olden days, elderly people generally enjoyed a high status. They were occupied with household activities and their grandchildren. They were considered and consulted in all family decisions. So, leisure time activities were not identified. But now the situation of elderly people has changed with industrialization, scientific progress, weakening of the joint family system, and emphasis on an individual's initiation and materialistic values. So, in recent years, leisure time has expanded markedly and the need for recreational activities for elderly people has increased.

Old age has a dual definition. It is the last stage in the life process of an individual, and it is an age group or generation comprising a segment of the oldest members of a population. The social aspects of old age are influenced by the relationship of the physiological effects of ageing and the collective experiences and shared values of that generation to the particular organization in which it exists. There is no universally accepted age that is considered old among or within societies. Often, discrepancies exist as to what age a society may consider old and what members in that society of that age and older may be considered old. Biologists, too, are not in agreement about the existence of an inherent biological cause for ageing. In most Western countries today, 60 or 65 is the age of eligibility for retirement and old age social programmes. However, many countries and societies regard old age as occurring anywhere from the mid-40s to the 70s.

There is no simple answer. In fact, there are several definitions and we tend to slip unknowingly from one to another. 'Old' is a powerful word in today's world. Old age is a major life change that alters one's relationship with the world around one, demanding new responses.

Old age is the closing period in the life span. It is the period when people 'move away' from previous, more desirable times of 'usefulness'. Like every other period in the life span, old age is characterized by certain physical and psychological changes. The effects of these changes determine, to a large extent, whether elderly men and women will make good or poor personal and social adjustments. The characteristics of old age, however, are far more likely to lead to poor adjustments than to good and to unhappiness rather than to happiness. That is why old age is dreaded even more today than middle age. The unfavourable social attitudes towards elderly people are reflected in the way the social group treats them, so it is not surprising that many elderly people develop unfavourable self-concepts.

Recreation is an art or experience selected by people during their leisure time to meet personal wants or desires, primarily for their own satisfaction. Since leisure is discretionary time, the quality of experience that takes place during this uncommitted period is within the determining power of each individual. This is of great importance for a free society, as the continued advance of its civilization depends increasingly on the ability of each individual to select leisure activities on the basis of quality. Conversely, in a totalitarian system of government, time is controlled by the state for its own benefit. The sophism of the 'All for the State' proposition becomes obvious because, finally, the individual is involved in a recreational experience and must find it meaningful because of the worth or feeling of accomplishment that it gives him.

The Meaning of Recreation

Recreation is viewed here as any activity or pursuit that is chosen voluntarily by participants in their leisure time, with the primary motivation of achieving personal pleasure and with a minimum of other hoped for goals or compulsions surrounding it. Clearly, when we refer to recreation as activity carried on for its own sake, it is difficult to ignore all the varied pressures one faces in making leisure choices. In considering recreation, an extremely broad range of possible characteristics must be recognized:

- Recreation may be the most trivial and unimportant of pursuits, or it may involve serious dedication and be on the highest level of purpose and intensity.
- It may involve a single casual episode, or it may continue as a deeply satisfying activity throughout a lifetime.
- It may be physically and mentally passive or require extremely active participation on a variety of levels.
- It may be completely solitary, or it may involve small groups or large masses of people.
- It includes all activities that are voluntarily chosen and pleasurable.

Therapeutic Recreation

Free time is a problem for many people. Some of us almost laugh at that statement for we all want more time to relax, to forget job hassles and responsibilities, and to have the opportunity to engage in our favourite activities and enjoy ourselves with our friends. But for many ill, handicapped and elderly people, free time is a major problem. The profession of therapeutic recreation deals with all aspects of such problems. As a profession, therapeutic recreation is rather new. It emerged during World War I, but had its greatest impact during World War II. During both wars, recreational activities were used with both physically disabled and psychologically disturbed soldiers and individuals in order to speed up the recovery process and help them adjust both to the treatment settings and to the communities to which they would be returning.

Therapeutic Recreation: A Process or a Service?

Perhaps the therapy versus recreation issue has resulted from attempts to define a therapeutic recreation service as a specific process, with most of the emphasis placed on therapeutic recreation rather than on service. Therefore, a therapeutic recreation service is defined as "a process which is utilized for purposive intervention in some physical, emotional and social behaviour to bring about a desired change in the behaviour and to promote the growth and development of the individual". One cannot accept the title of any profession to be a philosophical statement about a single specific process of service delivery. Therapeutic recreation identifies a type of service and utilizes many processes. The term, 'therapeutic recreation service', likewise identifies a population that needs or desires change that can be facilitated by the skills of a therapeutic recreation specialist. Within this total context, it is obviously important for elderly people to have a range of interesting and appropriate recreational opportunities made available to them, both to fill their long leisure hours and to meet, in a positive way, some of their important personal needs. What exactly are these needs and what contribution does recreation make to them? Five important contributions have been identified:

1. Improves physical health
2. Improves emotional well-being
3. Reawakens creative impulses
4. Provides meaningful roles
5. Offers a threshold for other services

Improves Physical Health

A number of studies have established that recreation of a physical nature makes a significant contribution to the physical condition of elderly people, particularly in terms of cardiac functions. Frequent moderate and enjoyable exercise means that people need not take drugs to release tension. It also helps to prevent unnecessary deterioration of the body and slows down the progressive breakdown of body systems. There is evidence that the satisfaction derived from accomplishment and continued physical activity is linked to human longevity. Dr Raymond Harris, a leading cardiologist, summed up the broad values of physical activities for elderly people, suggesting that exercise programmes should include four basic elements:

- Relaxation.
- Endurance exercises to condition the heart, lungs and circulation.
- Muscle strengthening exercises.
- Stretching exercises to improve joint mobility and reduce the aches and pains that accompany the ageing process.

Improves Emotional Well-Being

Meaningful involvement in social, physical and creative recreational activities tends to improve the state of mind of most elderly participants. It takes their minds off their preoccupation with themselves, their illnesses and their problems, and provides them with a sense of accomplishment. It generally contributes to a positive outlook on life.

Reawakens Creative Impulses

For many elderly people, the recreational programmes offered in old age homes or community based senior centres offer opportunities in art, music, theatre or literature, which awaken or revive creative impulses they may not have felt for years. Again, these stimulate intellectual functioning and emotional well-being and encourage a sense of vitality and energy. Obviously, recreation can provide an atmosphere conducive to developing friendships and to overcoming isolation and the resulting loneliness. For many elderly people, who have been widowed or divorced, such programmes may even result in friendships between the sexes that develop into marriage. There are a surprisingly large number of such marriages among elderly people who meet during recreational programmes. In institutional as well as community settings, recreation has been shown to have positive values in socialization. In a series of experimental studies across global from time to time by different scholars carried out in different state hospitals and nursing homes, it was demonstrated that such activities as swimming, arts and crafts, games and other social pastimes had a measurable positive effect on the social interaction patterns of elderly mental patients and residents.

Provides Meaningful Roles

As described earlier, an important need of many people is to play significant roles in society to supplement job or family responsibilities that have disappeared. For many elderly people, projects undertaken as a part of recreational programmes include giving assistance to the homebound or hospitalized and to children needing adult guidance. Some projects involve political campaigning, working to improve ecology or providing advice to minority group members who are beginning a business and need help from experienced, retired businessmen. The opportunity to contribute to society and to feel of real value to other human beings is of great importance to elderly people.

Offers a Threshold for Other Services

While recreation offers an important area of experience in itself for elderly people, it is also valuable in that it often paves the way for their making use of other vital social services. Elderly people often begin visiting a centre because of its recreational and social programmes. As they become aware of the other services it offers, such as health care, legal aid, budget planning and other advisory assistance, they tend to make use of them.

Places where Elderly People can Participate in Recreational Programmes

Recreational services are provided to elderly people in a variety of institutional and community settings:

- Senior citizens' centres and golden age clubs.
- Special residential centres such as leisure villages, retirement communities and special housing projects and residences for the 'well aged'.
- Day care programmes to serve elderly people who live at home, but have.
- Serious disabilities that require special supportive services

- Programmes for homebound elderly people.
- Geriatric units in hospitals or nursing homes or skilled nursing care facilities that serve dependent elderly people.

Recreational Needs and Elderly People

Elderly people in India face the predicaments that are peculiar to an increasingly industrialized and materialistic society and to cities that do not have enough space for their citizens. There are few open spaces earmarked for elderly people and their space within their homes is continually dwindling. Even as poor health catches up with them, they are faced with diminishing finances, social isolation, loneliness, excessive free time and loss of family and friends. In fact, the 60+ age group is the fastest growing in the country. Among elderly people, the growth rate of the 80+ age group is the highest. India will soon have the largest elderly population in the world. Yet, care for elderly people is amongst the youngest of 'causes' in India. Children's rights and women's rights, though relatively new, have been around for decades; but 'rights of the aged' is a nascent concept. It is subsumed under the Ministry of Social Welfare and ranked after women and children. Ageing is a time of multiple illnesses and general disability. Along with the biological changes, lifestyle factors are also important in treating disorders and diseases in old age. Old age diseases are not always curable, implying a strain on financial as well as physical health infrastructure resources, both at the macro and micro levels. However, feelings of well-being can still override actual physical discomfort if the surrounding environment is nurturing.

Aims of Community Recreation

Many policies, agencies, commissions and boards that guide a collative community approach to recreation prefer community recreation. Theoretically, these policies represent a series of broad goals intended to further the worthy use of leisure for all the people of the community. Some aims of such organized recreation programmes are:

- To contribute to a cultural heritage of a people committed to standards of beauty in society.
- To achieve a quality of leisure activity which sets a level for society and contributes ultimately to improving the lives of everyone.
- To enrich community living through opportunities for satisfaction of people's need of fellowship.
- To provide people with civic responsibilities and other opportunities to serve their fellow human beings.
- To allow for individual self-realization in physical well-being, reorganization, prestige, new adventures and emotional outlets.
- To enhance human relationships through a process of improvement of social skills, group experiences and a refinement of habits, attitudes and appreciations.
- To promote economic efficiency. Recreation can be a physical or mental change from work, which enables people to work better.

Raising the Level of Recreational Discrimination

Recreational agencies and their professional leaders aim to provide only those forms of recreation that are beneficial to an individual and to society. A Westchester study pointed out that the principal reason for the existence of recreation commissions, park commissions and other educational and welfare groups is to raise the recreational standards of individuals and of people collectively, and thus to elevate the total community. The agencies are supported and their programmes promoted because the community believes that the participants must come to appreciate better recreational forms. People tend to act in response to the levels of opportunity available to them, so they will read, perform or respond according to what is offered. The mass aspects of recreation are largely beyond local control and, therefore, outside the powers of recreational agencies on the community level. The real forte of these organizations lies in their obligation to improve quality pursuits.

Role of Home Scientists

Home scientists can play an important role in fulfilling the recreational needs of elderly people. As home scientists carry out fieldwork in nursing homes and old age homes, they get a chance to acquire information about the tendencies, needs and psychology of elderly people and learn how to treat them and work with them. During fieldwork, home scientists can help elderly people by writing letters for them or taking them to a place of worship or by just listening to them. They can remain in touch with them even after the fieldwork is completed. As home scientists know the psychology of elderly people, they can be more effective in treating their own grandparents and other elderly people in their community. Elderly people also need some recreational activities. Here are some suggestions for this:

- The state and society should give importance to elderly people and encourage them to visit places of worship or go out for walks.
- Day care centres should be started, where elderly people can meet and mingle with their peers and spend their time in a socially meaningful manner.
- Activities which are interesting and ensure adequate incentives should be planned so that elderly people can keep themselves busy and avoid loneliness.
- Policies and programmes should be framed keeping elderly people in mind.

Social Support

Social support provides recreational activities and a small contribution to assist with the cost of meals, transport and programme activities. Referrals may be made to the social support team leader or programme development officer. Social support groups can have:

- Social groups for older people.
- Arts, exercise and outdoor activities.
- Social programmes for those living in supported residential services.

- Organizing games and competitions such as Antakshari and *garba*.
- Improve muscular and bone strength.
- Lending libraries.
- Periodical religious discourses.
- Provide an opportunity for fun.
- Organizing talks by dietician.
- Improve joint flexibility.
- Walking groups.
- Organization of laughing clubs.
- Conducting Yoga camps.
- Performance of mythological plays.
- Arranging competitions such as debates, elocution, games, music and mimicry.
- Engaging them in fun activities with children, such as story telling.

Life Skills Empowerment

Various activities can be used to upgrade the skills and capacities of elderly people through a number of skill and personal development programmes, including life skills such as problem solving, self-awareness, communication, coping skills and decision making. Empowering individuals with such skills has been a continuous and specialized activity of the Department of Extension and Communication, Faculty of Family and Community Sciences, MS University of Baroda, in Vadodara.

Barriers

There are different barriers that limit the recreational activities of the 60+ population – scarce financial resources, lack of transportation, poor health, high fees and failure to get information being among them. At this age, they need more support, care and love.

Elderly people are generally not able to work very hard because they suffer from physical problems. So, they should be given activities like games that enable them to exercise their bodies and also entertain them. Weekly get-togethers, where they can chat and share their feelings with others, are a great idea. They can also be given short-term job opportunities, which enable them to work according to their interests and need. Different researches clearly shows that older people who engage in a variety of recreational activities are happier and derive more satisfaction from their lives. Lifelong educational experiences and leisure can possibly be given to elderly people because they have ample time and can be motivated to attain intrinsic goals from such educational experiences. Since educational activities may also help elderly people to recognize possibilities and opportunities they might otherwise miss, they may find continuing learning helpful after their retirement. Proper programmes are needed to provide such lifelong learning experiences. Regular physical activity can help elderly people maintain their vigour. Those who do sedentary activities are more likely to grow weak and ill than those who engage in moderate aerobic activities. People's motivation to engage in physical activity is based on three postulates: self-efficacy, outcome expectations, and self-evaluated satisfaction or dissatisfaction. We must remember elderly people also need recreation like any one else.

Our society will continue to boast of using chronological age for many purposes. We can live with this practice if we recognize that the setting up of a chronological checkpoint for calling a person 'old' is simply a matter of administrative or statistical convenience. It is an unfortunate use, but difficult to avoid. We can refuse to be swept along by the implicit relationship between chronological age and human values. Ideally, both sets of considerations should be taken into account. Problems arise when people are not given the opportunity to function as they are able to because of environmental restrictions. More awareness of these differing frameworks would help us develop flexible pathways through the entire lifespan of every human being. It will also help if we bear in mind the difference between ageing and being old. Ageing can be looked on as a process or set of processes. Oldness, however, is a state of the mind. We can set 'oldness' relatively late in life, and we can choose to regard it as a desirable or dreadful condition. At this age of their lives, elderly people need to be taken care of and made to feel special.

Bibliography

Astin, D.R. 1987. *Therapeutic Recreation Process and Techniques*. John Wiley & Sons, Canada, Quebec.

Butler, G. 1976. *Introduction to Community Recreation*. McGraw Hill Book Co., New York.

Chen, L., Pass, F.S. and Seidensticker, E. 2004. *Studies in Global Equality: Human Insecurity in a Global World*. Viva Books Pvt. Ltd., New York.

Murphy, J.E. 1987. *Recreational Cultural Activities in Social Education*. Indian Adult Education Association, New Delhi.

Nesbitt, J.A. and Brown, P.D. 1970. *Recreation and Leisure Services for the Disadvantaged*. Lea & Febiger, Philadelphia.

Webliography

gn.wikipedia.org/wiki/Recreation
http: //aja.co.in/serviccs.html
http: //india.gov.in/citizen/senior citizen/senior citizen.php
http: //www.recreativeresources.com/trbenefits.htm
http: //www.rho.org/html/definition_htm
http: //wwwjdictionary.net/recreation
www3.ngwberry.org/kl2maps/glossary/index.html

14 Recreation in Old Age Homes

Ageing is an important part of the human condition. It is a biological reality, which has its own dynamics, largely beyond human control. Ageing is defined differently in different societies. Ageing is a part of life. It begins with conception and terminates in death. The elderly people in a society are the people who have given their resources to the society and, once their resources are eroded, get pushed back by the society to its periphery.

In general, ageing is seen in two ways. First, it is described as an orderly and regularly process of change, or a gradually accelerating decline in the speed and precision of people's motor performance, learning and immediate recall. The somatic musculature begins to fatigue more easily and to recover more slowly after exertion (Cameron, 1945). Ageing is also seen as irregular, as a period of 'subtle variation'. It is not a simple slope down which everyone slides at the same speed. It is a flight of irregular stairs, down which some journey more quickly than others. This downward progress may be hastened or retarded by several factors, such as heredity, diseases, environment and past habits (Howell, 1953: 45).

Old age consist of ages nearing or surpassing the average life span of human beings and, thus, the end of the human life cycle. Ageing cannot be exactly defined because it does not have the same meaning in all societies. In many parts of the world, people are considered old because of certain changes in their social roles or activities; for example, people may be considered old when they become grandparents or when they begin to do less or different work. The age of 60 or 65, roughly equivalent to the retirement ages in most developed countries, is said to be the beginning of old age. In many parts of the developing world, chronological time has little or no importance in the meaning of old age. Other socially constructed meanings of age are more significant such as the roles assigned to older people; in some cases, it is the loss of their usual roles, accompanied by physical decline, which is significant in defining old age. Thus, in contrast to the chronological milestones that mark life stages in the developed world, in many developing countries, old age is seen to begin at the point when active contribution is no longer possible.

Late adulthood is the term coined by developmental psychologists to describe the period in an individual's life beginning at ages 60 or 70 and ending in death. At the moment, there is no United Nations standard numerical criterion, but the UN has agreed that the cut-off for referring to elderly population is 60+ years.

Status of Elderly People in India

The segment of the population that is aged 60 years and above is called the geriatric population. The phenomenon of population ageing (defined as increase in the median age of the population) is already a major social and health problem in developed countries. According to the 1991 Census of India, 6.3 per cent of the country's total population was geriatric. Over the decades, the geriatric population has been steadily increasing as a proportion of the total population. This rapid growth of the elderly population is a challenge to the medical profession, the administration and society. Elderly people suffer from a variety of problems, which are increasingly drawing the attention of the government and the public.

Most elderly people have retired from full time jobs. This means that their income is suddenly reduced. Economic hardships and the consequent lowered standards of living affect the body and the mind. Retirement, change in housing, and illness or death of a spouse greatly affect the physical well-being of elderly people. Their socio-economic problems are aggravated by lack of social security and inadequate facilities for health care, rehabilitation and recreation. In most developing countries, pensions and social security are restricted to those who have worked in the public sector or the organized sector of industry.

At this stage of life, people face a number of mental changes. These changes include memory impairment, rigidity of outlook and dislike of changing trends, especially sociocultural norms. They face social problems such as those caused by the breakup of the joint family system, nuclear families, housing shortages in urban areas, and the increasing participation of women in the workforce because women continue to be the health care providers for elderly people at the household level.

Elderly people suffer from various health problems that result from the ageing process, such as senile cataracts, glaucoma, nerve deafness, musculoskeletal changes affecting locomotion, failure of special senses and poor reflexes (resulting in accident proneness) and enlargement of the prostate gland in men. The most common diseases in this category are ischemic heart disease, hypertension, diabetes, cancer and respiratory diseases due to chronic bronchitis and emphysema. These are characterized by an increasing incidence of these conditions in a geometric or exponential fashion, as a function of age. Elderly people also suffer from conditions that are in the domain of psychological and psychosociological activity, which are caused by lowered living standards due to retirement and social maladjustment. While advances in science and technology have prolonged life expectancy, population ageing has brought about changes in cultural and social patterns, which have deprived elderly people of their social status, quality of life, self-esteem and of a chance to function usefully in society.

Status of India's Demographic Transition

One of the major features of demographic transition in the world has been the considerable increase in the absolute and relative numbers of elderly people.

India was in the first phase of transition till 1920, when both birth and death rates were high. At that time, the population of India was 251 million. The second phase of demographic transition started soon after 1920 and lasted up to 1971. During this period, decline in the death rate become sharper, especially during the 1940s and 1950s, while the birth rate remained quite high till 1961–71. The third phase of demographic transition started during the late 1970s, when the birth rate also started declining. This trend continued through the 1980s and it is expected that, in the next couple of decades, there will be faster declines in both the birth and death rates.

India will enter into the fourth phase of demographic transition by 2020 (Premi, 1991).

Demographic Profile of Elderly People in India

Elderly people are becoming a significant group in Indian society. Population ageing has received increasing attention in recent years, particularly in developing countries. This is a phenomenon characterized by decline in fertility levels and continued increase in life expectancy levels. These two variables are bringing about fundamental changes in the age structure of the population of societies in most parts of the world and these changes mark demographic transition. This transition outlines a shift from high levels of mortality and fertility to lower levels and is characterized by a rapid drop in mortality, followed by a somewhat slower decline in fertility.

India is gradually undergoing a demographic change as a result of many factors, including specific development programmes. India is a vast country both in terms of area and population. It has a total area of 3,288,000 square kilometres and its population was estimated to be around 1,027,015,247 on 1 March 2001. The total working population is estimated to be about one-third of this number. The dependency ratio is, therefore, around 1:2. Around 25.8 per cent of the population is reported to be living below the poverty line (Subramanya, 1994). According to the 1991 Census, India had 60 million elderly (60+) people. This is about 6.7 per cent of the total population, up from 5.97 per cent in 1971 and 6.32 per cent in 1981. The percentage of elderly people is much higher in rural areas (20.3%) than in urban areas (1.97%). The number of elderly people is likely to reach around 120 million by 2031 (EPW Research Foundation, 1994).

The size of the elderly population in India increased from 20 million in 1951 to 60 million in 2001 and is expected to climb to 107 million in 2010 and 198 million in 2050 (UN, 1995). In developed countries, where the demographic transition started earlier, the elderly population already forms a significant proportion of the total population, but in the developing countries, ageing issues have only recently begun to emerge as a cause of concern. This is because the proportion of and the number of elderly people in most of these countries are still quite low. In mid-1995, the world's elderly population (defined as 60+ people) was estimated at 542.7 million. One in every 11 of the world's inhabitants is at least 60 years of age. Around 55 per cent of the world's elderly people are women, underscoring their lower levels of mortality as compared to men. It is projected that Asia will have the majority of the world's elderly population by the turn of the 20th century.

The Jalaram Seva Samaj Trust

Old age leads to the retirement of elderly people from their occupations, their activities decrease due to their physical and mental disabilities, and they experience a void in their lives. Due to family circumstances, their desire to live their last days in peace and harmony with their near and dear ones is left unfulfilled. The perceived or actual decline in the feelings of their family members and their rude behaviour can make elderly people even more conscious of their dependence on others, leading to a further decline in their zest for life. Society and the government, too, neglect elderly people and what little is done is not enough. In such a situation, elderly people seek support. The presence of elderly people in a family, which earlier led to a sense of discipline, peace and pleasure, is unwelcome today. Wherever the fault may lie, the problem is commonly felt and a societal solution is needed.

An attempt in this direction was made by some philanthropists of Vadodara who believed in the maxim, 'Service to People is Service to God'. They got together at the initiative of the late Mr R.C. Gandhi, the late Mr Kamlashankar Pandya, and Mr J.D. Ray and started an old age home in August 1984. The old age home was started in a house of Navjivan Society, Ajwa Road, with seven people; this had increased to 61 at the time of the study. The house that was used for the old age home belonged to Mr Ray, who offered it for the purpose without charging any rent, but because it was located away from Vadodara city, there were some logistical problems, such as food arrangements. These were solved when the old age home was later shifted to a more central location within the city in Ashapuri Society, thanks to a trust, the Jalaram Seva Samaj Trust, set up by Mr Gandhi and his wife, Mrs Nirmalaben Gandhi, and the monetary donation of Rs 5 lakh that they made to it. Later, it was shifted once again, this time to Jalaram Seva Sadan in Nizampura.

The old age home sets out a busy timetable for its residents. They are served morning tea, lunch, afternoon tea and dinner. All, except the very ill or disabled, eat together, which fosters togetherness. Room service is provided for the very ill and the disabled. Individual tastes are kept in mind to a great extent. Care is taken to provide a balanced diet. The Jalaram Sevashram Trust provides food grains and groceries. Morning and evening prayers, religious discourses and bhajan *mandalis* are arranged regularly. Religious festivals are celebrated. Eminent people are invited from time to time to share their knowledge and experience with the residents.

Changes in the lifestyle of the younger generation have made the setting up of old age homes a necessity. Such homes provide a space for the older generation to live life at their own pace, on their own terms, and with their peer group. They are charged a nominal amount at these homes. They feel at home with people of their own age, who understand the stage of life that they are experiencing and who can help them and be helped by them.

Health care at the Jalaram Seva Sadan is provided by Positive Health Clinic, a homeopathic institution run by Dr Mukesh Batra. Regular diagnostic camps are organized with the help of S.S.G. Hospital and Yogini Vasantidevi Hospital in Vadodara. Mr Shashikant Sakarlal Velani takes care of the medical expenses. Currently, the old age home has 50 double rooms, with attached bathrooms. Each resident pays Rs 600 per month for one year. These residents belong to various nearby states and regions, such as Maharashtra, Saurashtra and Vadodara itself. The students of the Department of Extension and Communication, Faculty of Family and Community Sciences, MS University of Baroda, and Anand College go to the old age home for their fieldwork and also to help take care of the residents and to entertain them and spend time with them.

Social Aspects of the Elderly Residents of Jalaram Seva Sadan

Table 14.1 *Distribution by Sex of Residents at Jalaram Seva Sadan*

(N = 61)

Sex	*No.*	*Percentage (%)*
Females	32	52.46
Males	29	47.54

The above table shows that there are more women than men at the Sadan.

Table 14.2 *Distribution by Religion of Residents at Jalaram Seva Sadan*

(N = 61)

Religion	*No.*	*Percentage (%)*
Hindus	61	100

All the residents are Hindus.

Table 14.3 *Time Spent at Jalaram Seva Sadan by Residents*

(N = 61)

Time Duration	*No.*	*Percentage (%)*
0–3 Years	32	52.46
3–6 Years	18	29.51
6–9 Years	11	18.03

Nearly half of the residents have been living at the Sadan for less than three years. Only 18 per cent of them have lived there for six–nine years.

Table 14.4 *Distribution by Age of Residents at Jalaram Seva Sadan*

(N = 61)

Age	*No.*	*Percentage (%)*
Below 50 Years	03	04.92
51–60 Years	06	09.84
61–70 Years	21	34.43
71–80 Years	21	34.43
81–90 Years	08	13.11
Above 90 Years	02	03.28

An equal percentage of residents fall in the age groups of 61–70 years and 71–80 years (34.43 per cent each). A surprising 3 per cent of the residents have crossed the age of 90 years. The three people aged below 50 years are a couple and their son, who live at the Sadan and do the cooking and other work there.

Table 14.5 *Earlier Place of Residence of Residents at Jalaram Seva Sadan*

(N = 61)

Place of Residence	*No.*	*Percentage (%)*
Vadodara	49	80.33
Mumbai	05	08.20
Surat	03	04.92
Ahmedabad	01	01.64
Anand	01	01.64
Rajkot	01	01.64
Surendranagar	01	01.64

The majority – 80 per cent – of the residents at the Sadan are from Vadodara city. A small percentage – 8 per cent and 5 per cent – has come from Mumbai and Surat, respectively. There are also residents from Ahmedabad, Anand, Rajkot and Surendranagar.

The above tables show that people of different ages and sexes reside at the Jalaram Seva Sadan. However, they all share a religion.

Recreation Project for Elderly People

The students of the Department of Extension and Communication, Faculty of Family and Community Sciences, MS University of Baroda, in Vadodara, undertook a project at the Jalaram Seva Sadan.

Methodology

A schedule of activities was drawn up with different activities such as Yoga and talks on health tips for elderly people, art of living, acupressure, laughter therapy, successful ageing and fighting depression.

Activities under the Project

Expert Talk on Yoga

Yoga enables people to live a better life. Yoga can cure and protect them from many diseases and bring about mental peace. There are many *pranayams*, *asanas* and meditation techniques in Yoga that help alleviate both physical and mental ailments.

Objectives:

- To provide basic knowledge about Yoga to the residents
- To provide them some physical exercise
- To cure or alleviate their physical and mental ailments.

Activity: Kusum Pandya, an expert from Yoga Niketan in Fatehgunj, was invited to give a talk on basic Yoga. She explained the meaning of Yoga; its importance in our lives; the different types of Yoga; which types are suitable for elderly people; how, when and where to practise it; and points to be kept in mind while practising it. Teaching materials such as charts and posters with big, clear visuals were prepared to show the residents the various *asanas* and to create an environment of peace. Pamphlets brought in from Yoga Niketan were used during the talk. Students of Yoga Niketan demonstrated the various *asanas* during the talk. The residents of the Sadan were seen to participate with interest. Some of them posed questions to Ms Pandya.

Expert Talk on Elderly People and their Health

Health is a very important aspect of life, whether physical or mental. So, an expert talk on elderly people and their health was arranged and Ms Neelam and Ms Krishna Patel invited to give the talk. The topics covered in the talk included the dos and don'ts required to be followed at this time of life: drink water regularly, go for a small walk daily, avoid too many spices and salt in daily meals, etc. The two experts showed the residents the food pyramid and explained to them what quantities of each segment of the pyramid they should include in their daily meals. They also gave the residents some important guidelines to keep them healthy and fit both physically and mentally. The residents enjoyed the programme. They discovered the different activities that would keep them healthy.

Expert Talk on Art of Living

Art of Living and its concepts are very relevant to elderly people and can help them immensely in improving the quality of their lives. The expert talk on this topic was given by Mr Valjibhai Patel. Mr Patel stressed on the ways in which one could live a happy life. He told the residents that they should not live in their past, but focus on the present and think positively about it. Art of Living is all about accepting life in its totality and its motto is to 'only connect' – connect people across all communities and countries with love, to turn the tide of time by reviving human values and strengthening them. Art of Living helps to move beyond tolerance to unconditional acceptance and love. It teaches simple methods of achieving happiness in life by discovering one's beautiful inner self. It shows how to shed gloom, control all negative emotions such as anger, hatred, greed and lust, and be a positive person, no matter what the situation. The session helped the residents acquire information on Art of Living and how they could improve their outlook on life.

Expert Talk on Acupressure

Acupressure is a traditional Chinese medicine technique. It involves placing physical pressure using your fingers, hand or elbow, or with the aid of various devices, on the different acupuncture points on your body. Acupressure does not require the intake of any medicines, but it should be undertaken only under expert supervision. If done properly, it can help elderly people immensely in their routine life and alleviate all kinds of health problems.

Mr Dushant Modi, an qualify acupressure expert delivered the short, but useful, talk on acupressure to the residents of Jalaram Seva Sadan on 14 September 2007. In his talk, he gave information on small routine pressure points. He explained the pressure points on the hands and legs. A big chart with illustrations was prepared for the talk and handouts were distributed during it. The residents enjoyed the talk because they found it useful. They asked Mr Modi all kinds of questions.

Expert Talk on Laughter Therapy

Laughter is the best medicine, goes an old maxim, and it has been proved conclusively that laughter does help in keeping people healthy. Mr Trambak Joshi, a member of a local Laughter Club, gave the talk. Laughing can be equated with Yoga. It does not require any money or physical work and can be done easily by elderly people. Elderly people are usually very serious, so this is a good way of keeping them both entertained and healthy. The talk dwelt on basic laughter therapy and its advantages, with many examples of its good effects. Some of the points touched upon were:

- Live life happily.
- Do not bother about the past; live in the present.
- Be satisfied with what you have and don't expect anything from anyone.

At the end of the session, everyone joined together and sang a song. The talk was interesting and informative and the residents of the Sadan enjoyed it.

Expert Talk on Successful Ageing

Purnima Khanna visited the Sadan to give a talk on successful ageing on 18 October 2007. Ms Khanna works at the Women's Studies and Resource Centre at the MS University of Baroda in Vadodara. She talked about how elderly people should try and remain happy in this phase of their lives. Charts were prepared and used as teaching aids. The charts bore the points of discussion. Khanna covered health aspects, goals of life, coping capacity, creative expression, and spiritual, physical and emotional independence. First of all, there was an introductory session between the residents and Ms Khanna. Then she talked about healthy living and the positive effects of Yoga and exercise in maintaining good health. She told the residents that they could express their creativity by writing poems, stories and plays. She also discussed how they could cope with their problems. She ended the session with a song from an old Hindi film, *Hum Dono*, called *Main zindagi ka saath nibhata chala gaya*.

The residents of Jalaram Seva Sadan took a keen interest in all these expert talks and attended them regularly. They said they got to learn something new from the talks. They also enjoyed the more practical sessions on Yoga and acupressure and said these helped them to lead a more healthy physical and mental life.

Plays

Plays were performed at the Sadan for the entertainment of the residents and to inform them about different routine issues. Six plays were performed by the third year students of the Department of Extension and Communication on different topics such as literacy, good health and cleanliness. The humour, music and variety of characters in the plays made them interesting for the residents to watch. The residents found the puppet plays the most interesting because of their innovative value.

Bhavai

Folk media is a traditional medium of disseminating messages to people. It is a live folk art. The folk medium of *bhavai* was chosen as a medium for disseminating messages to the residents of Jalaram Seva Sadan.

A *bhavai* on *Anand Ashram No Vesh* was performed by the students of the Faculty of Performing Arts at the MS University of Baroda. It was performed under the guidance of Mr Rajul Mehta, senior lecturer at the Faculty. The *bhavai* focused on enjoying the last phase of life. It had two parts. The first part showed elderly people going to an old age home of their own free will; the second part showed them having to go to an old age home because of their family circumstances.

The *bhavai* was made more humorous and interesting with the use of traditional vocal instruments. It was full of music and entertainment. The residents enjoyed the *bhavai* and related to the characters in it.

Antakshari

An Antakshari session was organized for elderly people by the senior MSc students of the Department of Extension and Communication. Slips of paper carrying Hindi words such as *kajal*, *choodi*, *dupatta* and *zindagi* were prepared. The rules of the game were simple. Music was played and a parcel had to be passed around among the residents. When the music stopped, the person who was left holding the parcel had to pick a slip of paper and sing a song on the theme given on it. This game was planned in accordance with the interests of the residents. Liveliness was maintained throughout the game and it was ensured that none of the residents got bored.

Garba

Garba is a popular folk dance form of Gujarat, which is danced during the Navaratri festival. The nine days of the festival are celebrated with a lot of energy and enthusiasm and is popular among all age groups. From the spiritual point of view, elderly people wait for this festival. So, a *garba* was planned by the students at the Sadan on the first day of Navaratri. The students wore the traditional *garba* costumes. Initially, some of the female residents were reluctant to participate in the *garba*, but once the students began dancing, they also joined in.

Conclusion

The status of elderly people in India is a cause of worry. They suffer from health, economic and social problems. They have performed their duties and carried out their responsibilities in life, but are now ignored by the people around them and looked upon as a burden. In spite of still having many abilities and capabilities, they are not given an opportunity to utilize their time in a constructive manner. All these factors lead to feelings of depression in elderly people. They need encouragement to live happy lives. The establishment of old age homes has contributed to helping elderly people lead healthy and peaceful lives. In these homes, they are treated well and given the opportunity to enjoy their lives to the fullest. They are in a familial environment and with people who have suffered similar problems. This improves their physical and mental health to a great extent.

Our journey to the Jalaram Seva Sadan was an enriching experience. We got to know the status of the residents of this old age home. We found that the programmes that we arranged for them were quite successful. Such programmes, especially those that involve them as well, should be conducted at regular intervals to entertain and enlighten elderly people.

Elderly people are the backbone of our nation. We should be grateful to them for the positive contributions they have made to our lives and our society. Caring for their interests and recreation when they are old and retired is the duty of not just their families or an institution, but of everyone in society.

Bibliography

Bond, John, Coleman, P. and Peace, Sheila. 1993. *Ageing in Society*. Sage Publications, New Delhi.

Irvin, Boscow. 1969. *Social Integration of the Aged*. Collier Macmillan Free Press, Canada, Toranto.

Kohli, A.S. 1999. *Social Situation of the Aged in India*. Anmol Publications Pvt. Ltd., New Delhi.

Tharabhai, L. 2002. *Ageing: Indian Perspective*. Decent Books, New Delhi.

Webliography

http://india.gov.in/citizen/senior_citizen/policies_schemes.php

http://india.gov.in/citizen/senior_citizen_08-06-07/policies_schemes.php

http://socialjustice.nic.in/social/sdcop/opersons.htm

http://www.helpageindia.org/

http://www.nios.ac.in/secpsycour/unit-14.pdf

http://www.webmed.com/

http://www.whoindia.org/EN/Section20/Section26.htm

15 Health and Recreation for Institutionalized Elderly People

Human beings pass through various stages during their lifetime: infancy, childhood, adolescence, adulthood and old age. The biological transition through these different stages has cultural and human overtones because age definition and differentiation carry significance at both the society and individual levels. At the society level, they function as indicators for the allocation of various roles and functions. At the individual level, they serve as an important base for self-perception and role performance.

Ageing is a natural process, but old age is arbitrary. Getting old is the result of the interplay of biological, social, psychological and ecological factors. Old age is the ultimate phase of the human cycle, and the timing of this phase, its impact on role relationships, and the meaning attached to it vary in different societies and even in different subways of a society.

In traditional Indian society, elderly people held positions of supremacy in the family and society and were endowed with special privileges. It was conventionally believed that wisdom blossomed with advancing age, so elderly people, with their rich, diversified life experiences, were in a better position to guide the younger generation in most matters. In traditional Indian culture, old age was considered a stage of human development in which people attain wisdom, maturity and social and economic stability with social recognition and emotional fulfilment, leading to the last phase of life – spiritual salvation. Elderly people were the most respected in the family and the centre of authority. All the decisions pertaining to the family were made by them. They enjoyed great respect in society.

However, this situation is now changing fast because of the effects of rapid industrialization, urbanization and population pressure on the family. Family patterns are changing from joint and extended families to nuclear families, and this has increased the problems of elderly people. Their adult children have other family responsibilities and are unable to look after them; sometimes, adult children have migrated and are no longer around to look after them.

Demographic and Socio-economic Influences

The ageing of a population is an obvious consequence of the process of demographic transition. This chapter presents details of the various dimensions of the life of elderly people in old age homes. The shadow of life is lengthening in Indian society – there were around 77 million people aged above 60 in the country in 2001, up from 19 million in 1951. With life expectancy going up continually thanks to advances in medical care and improvements in quality of life, and with birth rates falling, elderly people constitute the fastest growing segment of society.

A greater degree of financial insecurity resulting from inadequate financial resources is seen to be a major problem with elderly people in India. Loss of economic independence seems to be correlated to increase in age. People who are self-employment are compelled to continue working as long as they can because of economic necessity. They need social assistance and support in their old age.

The social aspects of old age are influenced by the relationship of the physiological effects of ageing and the collective experiences and shared values of that generation to the particular organization of the society in which they exist. In agrarian societies, elderly people enjoy a status of respectability. Their life experiences and knowledge are regarded as valuable, especially in preliterate societies, where knowledge is orally transmitted. The range of activities in these societies allows elderly people to continue to be productive members of their communities. Familial relationships tend to be the focus of elderly people's attention. However, with the recent changes in the family structure – from several generations living in close proximity to self-contained nuclear families of only parents and young children – older people have become isolated from the younger generation. This is causing several physical and psychological health problems among elderly people.

Physical and Psychological Health Problems

When people reach the threshold of old age, their bodily systems become increasingly less efficient and less resistant to disease. Consequently, the general belief prevailing in our society that ailments are a part of growing old. Cognitive impairment may cause functional problems for elderly people. The physiological effects of ageing differ widely from individual to individual. However, chronic ailments, especially aches and pains, are more prevalent than acute ailments, requiring older people to spend more time and money on medical problems than younger people.

Psychological well-being is an equally important aspect of health. Like other human beings, elderly people also have various psychological problems, such as memory impairment, depression, insomnia, fear, anxiety, social maladjustment and insecurity. These problems may stem from both physiological and social factors. Many elderly people face significant life changes and stressors that put them at risk for depression. Those at the highest risk include older adults with a personal or family history of depression, failing health, substance abuse problems, or inadequate social support. The causes of and risk factors that contribute to psychological problems in elderly people include:

- *Loneliness and isolation:* Living alone; dwindling social circle due to deaths or relocation; decreased mobility due to illness or loss of privileges
- *Reduced sense of purpose:* Feelings of purposelessness or loss of identity due to retirement or physical limitations on activities
- *Health problems:* Illness and disability; chronic or severe pain; cognitive decline; damage to body image due to surgery or disease

- *Medication:* Many prescription medications can trigger or exacerbate depression
- *Fears:* Fear of death or dying; anxiety over financial problems or health issues
- *Bereavement:* The loss of a spouse or partner; the deaths of friends, family members and pets.

Among the factors that precipitate emotional problems are loneliness, poor health, loss of income and the death of a spouse or close friends. Any one of these causes can lead to depression. Preoccupation with one's health, social inertia, feelings of helplessness, lack of interest, sadness, lack of sleep or a tendency to oversleep, self-pity, loneliness, lack of appetite and boredom are common problems and could all indicate the onset of depression. The rising cost of medical care has caused growing concern among elderly people and societies, in general resulting in constant revaluation and reform of institutions and programmes designed to aid elderly people with these expenses. Certain aspects of sensory and perceptual skills, muscular strength and certain kinds of memory tend to diminish with age, rendering older people unsuitable for some activities.

Old age is seen as the time of life when one's health deteriorates progressively, so it is to be expected that a large proportion of older people will see themselves as being in poor health. The health status of elderly people is usually defined either by the presence or absence of disease as by the assessment of functional capacity. However, there is no denying that many of them are more susceptible to falling ill. Yet, it is surprising that while society considers old age a synonym of sickness, there is no such disease as old age. Life today has expanded in historically unprecedented proportions, greatly increasing the number of people who survive over the age of 65. Therefore, the instances of medical problems associated with ageing, such as certain kinds of cancer and heart disease, have increased, giving rise to greater consideration, both in research and social programmes, for accommodating this increase.

Why Society Needs Old Age Homes

India is a land rich in traditions, customs and culture. Indians were known for their respect and love for their elders. The parent-child bond was considered most sacred in India. When children entered school, the first thing they were taught was a verse from the *Taittiriya Upanishad*: "*Matru devo bhava, Pitru devo bhava; Acharya devo bhava, Atithi devo bhava* (May you be one who worships your mother, father, teacher and guests as God)." Parents make many sacrifices in bringing up their children and helping them attain good positions in life. Under Indian tradition and culture, it is the duty of a son to look after his parents. In olden days, people used to live together in joint families. Now, Indian society is changing rapidly as are its moral values. Many children do not, or cannot, look after their elderly parents, who live alone or in old age homes.

Status of Old Age Homes in India

The ambition of people all over the world to live long is now becoming reality due to their socioeconomic development and advances in science, particularly medical science. In India, around 7.5 per cent of the population is aged above 60 years and life expectancy is increasing gradually. Old age was never a problem in India. Old age homes were an alien concept and abuse of elderly people was considered a Western problem. Now, with the increase of life expectancy from 41 years in 1951 to 64 years today, hundreds of old age homes have sprung up in India. Neglect of parents has become a big issue, so much so that the Indian government has presented before Parliament the Maintenance and Welfare of Parents and Senior Citizens Bill 2006, which makes it mandatory for adult children to look after their parents.

As of 1998, there were 728 old age homes in India. Detailed information about 547 of these is available. Out of these, 325 homes are free of cost, 95 are 'pay and stay' homes, and 116 homes have both free and pay and stay facilities. A total of 278 old age homes in the country cater to the sick and disabled and 101 are exclusively for women.

As the role of families as a social safety net for elderly people is fast eroding, the poor among the elderly have become the most vulnerable section of society in India. The Indian government is waking up to meet this challenge head on. At present, more than 500 non-governmental organizations (NGOs) have been given grants-in-aid to provide services such as old age homes, day care centres and medical facilities for elderly people. The Delhi based International Federation on Ageing has been campaigning for free health care for senior citizens; decrease in the age limit for pension; a bigger, respectable living allowance; change in the eligibility criteria so that even if the combined family income is Rs 8,000, senior citizens are entitled to pension, creation and implementation of a social security scheme, and so on. It is irrefutable that old age homes are a necessity today because younger people do not have the time or, in many cases, the resources to meet their needs such as medical expenses and special food. But old age homes should be considered only as a secondary option. Elderly people are an asset in the family. They can impart much needed ethical values and code of conduct to the younger generation. Old age homes should be considered an option only for the betterment of elderly people by way of better physical and mental status and greater possibility for social bonding. For no reason should elderly people be made to feel that they are a burden. Builders could consider allocating a few houses within integrated townships at concessional rates to elderly people so that feelings of isolation go away, while proximity to dear ones is maintained.

Adult Education Programme at Swami Premdas Jalaram Old Age Home

This section gives details of the adult education programme, conducted by graduate students of Home Science Extension at the Swami Premdas Jalaram Old Age Home, Warsiya, Baroda, Gujarat.

Report on Institution

The Swami Premdas Jalaram Old Age Home is attached to the Swami Premdas Jalaram Hospital. This is a socio-economic organization that has been striving for the welfare of the poor, the needy, women and elderly people for the last 20 years. Swami Premdas (1940's) was the 11th *mahant* of a spiritual, religious and social mission in Sindh, in Pakistan. His principles were simplicity and service, purity and prayer. He used to run a free medical dispensary in his village, which served not only his own village, but also many other villages around it. He helped many mentally retarded people to regain their mental faculties with medicines and prayers. After the partition of India, Swami Premdas moved to Vrindaban in 1948. There, he set up an ashram, called Tulsi Nivas. In 1953, he moved to Vadodara. Swami Premdas believed firmly that service to mankind was the real worship of God. In 1988, he inaugurated the Swami Premdas Seva Niketan, which renders economic, educational, health and social services to the poor, the needy, women and elderly people. Later, the hospital, a medical research centre and the old age home were set up under the Swami Premdas Seva Niketan.

All these institutions focus on economic, educational, health and social services for the poor, the needy, women and elderly people. The old age home was inaugurated with the objective of providing health and recreational facilities to elderly people who are neglected by their own families and to enable them to live out the last years of their lives in dignity and comfort.

Facilities at the Old Age Home

The Swami Premdas Jalaram Old Age Home is a residential old age home, which receives funds from individual donors and a social defence grant. The monthly charge for use of services and facilities is Rs 650. The criteria for entry to the old age home are:

- The person should be aged 60 years or above.
- He should be self-dependent.
- He should be free from any kind of serious ailment.
- He should be able to take care of himself.

Methodology

The objective of the adult education programme was to conduct activities based on the needs and interests of the residents of the home. The fieldwork was assigned to the 2008–09 batch of MSc students of the Department of Extension and Communication,

Faculty of Family and Community Sciences, MS University of Baroda, in Vadodara. The aim was to enable the students to gain practical knowledge and experience of the adult education programme, which was constituted under the Lifelong Education Programme. The Swami Premdas Jalaram Old Age Home was selected for the fieldwork. The methodology was divided thus:

1. Planning of activities (Antakshri, passing the parcel, Garba etc.).
2. Construction of questionnaire.
3. Collection of data.

Construction of Questionnaire

A questionnaire for data collection was developed. It was divided into two sections:

Section I	Profile of the residents background information.
Section II	Perceptions of the residents regarding the services provided at the home.

Collection of Data

The data was collected using the interview schedule and observation schedule methods.

Findings and Observations

This section gives the details of the findings from the data that was collected with the help of the questionnaire as well as the case studies of the residents.

Table 15.1 *Percentage Distribution of Residents by Sex*

(N = 22)

Sex	*Percentage (%)*
Males	63.63
Females	36.36

This shows that more than 60 per cent of the residents are men and less than 40 per cent – 36.36 per cent – are women.

Table 15.2 *Percentage Distribution of Residents by Age*

(N = 22)

Age	*Percentage (%)*
Above 60 Years	18.18
Above 70 Years	54.54
Above 80 Years	18.18
Above 90 Years	9.09

Half of the residents at the old age home were in the age group of more than 70 years. An equal percentage – 18.18 per cent each – was aged above 60 years and above 80 years. Only 9.09 per cent of the residents were older than 90 years.

Table 15.3 *Percentage Distribution of Residents by Religion*

(N = 22)

Religion	*Percentage (%)*
Hindu	86.36
Sindhi	13.63

Most of the residents at the old age home – 86.36 per cent – were Hindus; a few – 13.63 per cent – were Sindhi.

Table 15.4 *Percentage Distribution of Residents by Marital Status*

(N = 22)

Marital Status	*Percentage (%)*
Married	18.18
Unmarried	13.07
Widow	36.37
Widower	31.09

Around 36.37 per cent of the residents were widows; 31.09 per cent were widowers. Only 18.18 per cent had been married; 13.07 per cent were unmarried.

Table 15.5 *Percentage Distribution of Residents by Education*

(N = 22)

Educational Status	*Percentage (%)*
Illiterate	12.5
Primary School	50.00
Secondary School	37.5

Exactly 50 per cent of the residents had been educated only up to the primary school level. Around 37.5 per cent of them had had secondary school education. Very few of them – 12.5 per cent – were illiterate.

Table 15.6 *Percentage Distribution of Residents by Family Type*

(N = 22)

Type of Family	*Percentage (%)*
Joint Family	25
Nuclear Family	75

The majority of the residents – 75 per cent – belonged to nuclear families; only 25 per cent came from joint families.

Table 15.7 *Percentage Distribution of Residents by Occupation*

(N = 22)

Occupation	*Percentage (%)*
Business	26.31
Service	36.84
Housewife	31.57
Unemployed	5.26

More than 30 per cent – 36.84 per cent – of the residents had been in service before they came to the old age home. Around 31 per cent had been housewives. More than 20 per cent – 26.31 per cent – had been in business. Very few of them – 5.26 per cent – had been unemployed.

Table 15.8 *Percentage Distribution of Residents by Duration of Stay at the Home*

(N = 22)

Duration	*Percentage (%)*
6–12 Months	23.52
1–5 Years	52.94
6–10 Years	5.88
11–15 Years	10.52
16–20 Years	5.88

More than half of the residents – 52.94 per cent – had been living in the old age home for one–five years and less than 25 per cent – 23.52 per cent – had been living there for the last 6–12 months. Around 10.52 per cent had been living in the home for 11–15 years. Only 5.88 per cent had been living there for 16–20 years.

Table 15.9 *Percentage Distribution of Residents by Reference for the Home*

(N = 22)

Reference for Old Age Home	*Percentage (%)*
Self	47.36
Children	21.05
Relatives	26.31
Friends	5.26

Less than half of the residents – 47.36 per cent – had come to the old age home of their own volition. More than 25 per cent – 26.31 per cent – had come because their relatives had referred them there. Around 21.05 per cent had been referred by their children; 5 per cent had been referred by friends.

The majority of the residents – 70.58 per cent – were meeting their expenses at the old age home with assistance from relatives. Less than 20 per cent – 17.64 per cent – were meeting their expenses with their own savings. Very few of them – 11.76 per cent – were using their pensions to meet their expenses.

Table 15.10 *Percentage Distribution of Residents by Source for Meeting Expenses*

(N = 22)

Source for Meeting Expenses	*Percentage (%)*
Personal Savings	17.64
Pension	11.76
Assistance from Relatives	70.58

Table 15.11 *Percentage Distribution of Residents by Health Problems*

(N = 22)

Diseases	*Percentage (%)*
Dental Problems	7.69
Joint Pains	53.84
Blood Pressure Problems	30.76
Headaches	15.38
Diabetes	7.69
Acidity	15.38
Back Pain	38.46

More than half of the residents – 53.84 per cent – said they suffered joint pains. Around 38.46 per cent said they had back pain. Some 30 per cent said they faced blood pressure problems; only 15.38 per cent said they suffered headaches and acidity. Very few of them – 7.69 per cent – reported they had diabetes.

Table 15.12 *Percentage Distribution of Residents by their Opinion on Home vs Old Age Home*

(N = 22)

Better Place	*Percentage*
Old Age Home	61.53
Home	38.46

The majority of the residents – 61.53 per cent – said they found the old age home a better place to live in; around 38.46 per cent said they would prefer to live at home.

Description of the Swami Premdas Jalaram Old Age Home

At present, there are 25 elderly people living in the Swami Premdas Jalaram Old Age Home. The home can accommodate 30 people in its five rooms. The men are grouped six to a room, while the women are put three to a room. The women residents have a toilet attached to their rooms, while the men have to use the common toilet.

As discussed earlier, the old age home is attached to the Swami Premdas Jalaram Hospital, so all the medical care and expenses are taken care of. No extra charge is taken from the residents for treatment or medication. Regular health check-ups are organized. Yoga classes are conducted daily on the lawns of the home, from 6.30 am to 7.30 am.

Simple, nutritious, vegetarian food is served in the common dining hall. The residents are provided two meals in a day – lunch at around 12.30 pm and dinner at around 7.30 pm. Water, including drinking water, is available 24 hours. Hot water for bathing is provided only in winter.

The residents pay the home Rs 650 per month. This amount can be paid monthly or in advance, as they choose. There is no special meeting place available at the home. The residents can meet their children or relatives in their rooms or in the common room.

According to their experience, the residents say that some of the other residents are friendly and share their feelings with them, while some others are narrow minded and very aggressive.

Recreational Facilities

The Swami Premdas Jalaram Old Age Home has a common hall in which all the recreational activities are conducted. It has a library from where the residents can borrow books. There is also a television set, a radio and an audio-cassette player. Indoor games such as Antakshari and Passing the Parcel are played. Picnics are arranged periodically to different religious places and to parks and gardens. Birthday celebrations are arranged at a nearby temple, where the priest garlands them and gives them flowers and his blessings. The various festivals are celebrated with gifts and feasts. Religious discourses are arranged from time to time. Religious leaders, philosophers and educationists are invited to the home to give educative, informative and positive information on various topics, including health and nutritious food.

Observations

- Most of the residents were interested in spiritual activities. Many of them participated enthusiastically on the day when spiritual activities were organized.
- They were eager to share their life experiences, whether happy or bitter, with others because they like to talk and they want somebody to listen to them.
- Only a few of them were not interested in participating in the different activities of the adult education programme.
- A few of them were interested in attending the programme, but not able to participate in the activities because of various physical problems.
- They reported that they did not get a chance to participate in any recreational activities at the old age home and that they waited eagerly for the students to visit.
- They participated enthusiastically in the games and said that they liked to play indoor games.

Bibliography

Arora, M. and Chadha, N.K. 1995. 'Social Support and Life Satisfaction of Institutionalized Elderlies', in *Indian Journal of Gerontology*, 9 (3 & 4), pp. 74–82.

Bakshi, R., Rajneesh, P. and Sandhu, P. 2002. 'Level of Satisfaction Derived by the Aged Living with Families and in Senior Citizen Homes', in *Indian Psychological Review 58*, No. 1, p. 1420.

Bali, A. 1997. 'Why Focus on Elderly Females?', in Kalyan Bagchi (ed.): *Elderly Females in India: Their Status and Suffering*. Society for Gerontological Research and Help Age India, New Delhi, pp. 36–7.

Cherian, J. 2003. 'Adjustment of the Elderly in Relation to Living Arrangements, Gender and Family Life Satisfaction', in *Indian Journal of Gerontology*, 17 (1 & 2), pp. 99–108.

Chittibabu, S.V. 1997. 'Value Orientation of Education'. Convocation address in *University News*, Vol. 35, No. 18, New Delhi, May.

Dave, Janak. 1997. *Bal Natak Digdarshankala*. Lakshmi Pustak Bhandar, Ahmedabad.

Dave, R.H. et al. (eds). 1986. *Learning Strategies for Post Literacy and Continuing Education in China, India, Indonesia, Nepal, Thailand and Vietnam*. Vol. 1.

Emine, G., and Emine, O. 2005. *Quality of Life Satisfaction: Perspective of Institutionalized Elderly Women and Men in Turkey*, Vol. 53, No. 7.

Goran, Hedebro. 1982. *Communication and Social Change in Developing Nations: A Critical View*. Iowa State University Press.

Hirway, I. 2000. 'Dynamics of Development in Gujarat: Some Issues', in *Economic and Political Weekly*, Vol. 35, Issues 35 & 36.

Mukhopadhya, Durgadas. 1978. *Lesser Known Forms of Performing Arts in India*. Sage Publications Delhi.

Mussan, P., Hozik, M.P. and Eichom, H. 1982. 'Early Adult Antecedents of Life Satisfaction at Age 70', in *Journal of Gerontology*, 37, pp. 316–22.

Pai, Reshma. 2000–01. 'Comparative Study of Effectiveness of Two Communication Media in Teaching Selected Aspects of Street Plays to the Students of Faculty of Home Science' (M.Sc. thesis). MS University of Baroda, Vadodara.

Paintal, A.C. 1997. 'Towards Value Education'. Convocation address in *University News*, Vol. 35, No. 6.

Pandya, Madhvi. 1993. 'Relative Effectiveness of Two Selected Strategies, Namely Live Programme vs Videoed Programme of Bhavai and Exhibition cum Demonstration for Promotion of Solar Cookers'. Ph.D. thesis, MS University of Baroda, Vadodara.

Parmer, Shyam. 1994. *Traditional Folk Media in India*. Research Press, New Delhi, 2nd edition.

Prakash, I.J. 1997. 'Women and Aging', in *Indian Journal of Economic Psychology*, 7 (4), pp. 425–46.

Satya Raju, R. 1997. 'Human Values in University Management', in *University News*, Vol. 35, No. 45, November.

Bibliography

Alur, M. 2002. *Invisible Children: A Study of Policy Exclusion*. Vivak Books Pvt. Ltd., New Delhi.

Ambekar, J.B. 1991. 'Communication and Rural Development', in *Social Change,* Vol. 21, No. 3, September.

Anandalakshmy, S. 1982. *Cognitive Competence in Infancy*. Indian Council of Social Science Research, New Delhi.

Antognoli, Paula T. 2000. 'Parent Child Relationship, Family Structure and Loneliness among Adolescents'. Ph.D. thesis, Texas Women's University.

Attarchand, A. 1987. *Poverty and Underdevelopment: New Challenges*. Gauri Publishing House, Delhi.

Balakrishna, S. 1983. 'Management Information System for Integrated Rural Development Programme', in *Yojana* 27(22).

Bali, A.P. 1996. 'Well-Being of Elderly: Social Change', in *Development Index,* Delhi, pp. 64–76.

Beltran, Luis Ramiro. 1978. 'Rural Communities in Developing Countries: The Prospects of Communication', in *Issues in Communication, No. 2*. International Institute of Communications, London.

Bibby, C. 2001. *Sex Education*. A.P.H. Publishing Corp., New Delhi.

Bucher, Charles A. 1985. *Administration of School Health and Physical Education Programme*.

Carney, Jan and Lauderdale, Denise. 1978. *Implementing Comprehensive School Health*. Macmillan Publishing Co. Inc., New York.

Census of India. 1991, 2001. Ministry of Information and Broadcasting, Government of India, New Delhi.

Census of India. 1991. 'Ageing Population of India: Analysis of the 1991 Census Data'. Registrar General of India.

Centre for Policy Research. 1983. *Population, Poverty and Hope.* Utpal Publishing House, New Delhi.

Centre on Integrated Rural Development for Asia and the Pacific. 1984. Workshop report on 'Multi-Level Information System for Integrated Rural Development'. Dhaka. June.

Chakraborty, B.G. 2003. 'North Bengal Small Growers', in *Contemporary Tea Time,* Vol. XII, No. 2, July-August, pp. 60–1.

Chakravarthy, Nikhil. 1995. 'Mahatma Gandhi: The Great Communicator', in *Mainstream,* April 8.

Chalkley, Alan. 1980. 'Development Journalism: A New Dimension in the Information Process', in *Media Asia* 7(4).

Chandra, K. and Dave, C. 2006. A Study of Insecurities in Senior citizens of Udaipur City', in *Social Welfare,* 53(1), pp. 32–36.

Chandrashekhar, S. 1950. *India's Population: Fact and Policy.* Indian Institute for Population Studies, Annamalai University, Tamil Nadu.

Chaube, S.P. 1964. *A Textbook for Pupil Teachers.* Vinod Pustak Mandir, Agra.

Chawla, N.L. 2002. 'Communication for Development', in *Mainstream* 24(16).

Clinard, M.K. 1981. *Statistics.* Ministry of Social Welfare, New Delhi.

Clinebell, Howard J. 1956. *Understanding and Counselling the Alcoholic.* Abingdon Press, New York.

Crickman, R.D. 1976. 'Community Communication Patterns', in M. Kochen and J.C. Donahue (eds): *Information for the Community.* American Library Association, Chicago.

Curran, James and Gurevitch, Michael. 1996. *Mass Media and Society.* Arnold, London.

Dalzell, A.J. 1975. *A Text Book of Health Education.* Tavistock Publications, London.

Dantwala, M.L. 1985. 'Garibi Hatao: Strategy Options', in *Economic and Political Weekly,* March 16.

Davies, Brian Meredith. 1977. *Community Health and Social Services.* Hodder & Stoughton, London.

Dey, Pradip Kumar. 1993. *Perspectives in Mass Communication.* Kalyani Publishers, New Delhi.

Dhillon, H.S., and Tolsma, D. 1992. 'Meeting Global Health Challenges: A Position Paper on Health Education'. International Union for Health Education and the Division of Health Education, WHO, Geneva.

Diaz, Bordenave, and Juan, E. 1977. *Communication and Rural Development.* UNESCO, Paris.

Dickinson, George E. 2000. 'Changing Religious Behaviour of Adolescents', in *Youth and Society*, Vol. 13, pp. 283–8.

Doron, Harold F. 1963. 'World Population Growth', in Philip Houser (ed.): *The Population Dilemma.* Columbia University.

Edward, M. and David, H. 1995. *Non-Government Organizations: Performance and Accountability, Beyond the Magic Bullet.* Earthscan Publications, London.

Elliott, Daphne S. 1967. *Health Education Patterns for Teaching.* Macmillan and Co. Ltd., London.

Elliott, Mabel A. and Merrill, Francis E. 1950. *Social Disorganisation.* Harper & Brothers, New York.

Encyclopaedia of HIV/AIDS: Problems and Control. 2007. Anmol Publication Pvt. Ltd., New Delhi.

Encyclopaedia of the Social Sciences: Index to Public Education, Health and Welfare. 1997. The Macmillan Co., New York, Vol. VIII.

European Centre for Leisure and Education. 1973, 1974. 'Adult Education and Changes in the Way of Life'. Paper presented at the Experts' Meeting of the Socialist Countries, Prague, 19–23 November. Printed in *Society & Leisure* (bulletin for sociology of leisure education and culture), No. 2.

Evans, David R. 1979. *Games and Simulations in Literacy Training.* IIALM, Tehran.

Farrington, J. and Lewis, D. 1993. *Non-Government Organizations and the State in Asia: Rethinking Problems in Sustainable Agriculture Development.* Routledge Publications, New York, pp. 1–37.

Faure, Edgar, and others. 1972. *Learning to Be: The World of Education Today and Tomorrow.* UNESCO.

Fawcett, James T. 1999. *Psychology Perspectives on Population*. Basic Books I.N.G. Publisher, New York.

Feiring, Williams Jesse and Shaw, Fannie B. 1966. *Methods and Materials of Health Education*. The Ronald Press Co., New York.

Fordham, Paul (ed.). 1985. *One Billion Illiterates, One Billion Reasons for Action: Report and Extracts from Papers of an International Seminar on Co-operation for Literacy*. International Council for Adult Education, West Berlin, Toronto.

Fowler, A. 2000. *The Virtuous Spiral: A Guide to Sustainability for Non-Government Organizations in International Development*. Earthscan Publications, London.

Freire, Paulo. 1972. *Pedagogy of the Oppressed*. Penguin, Harmondsworth.

Fuller, Richard C. and Myres, Richard R. 1991. 'The Natural History of a Social Problem', in *American Sociological Review*.

Gachuhi, D. and Matiru B. (eds). 1989. *Handbook for Designing and Writing Distance Education Materials*. Science and Documentation Centre, German Foundation for International Development Education, Bonn.

Gandhi, R. D. and Parmar D.T. *'Bibliography for Taluka Level Information'*. Ahmedabad, India: Gujarat Institute of Area Planning, (1977).

Ganesh S. 1995. *Lectures of Mass Communication*. Indian Publishers Distributors, Delhi.

Gardner, Ella. 1960. *Handbook for Recreation*. US Department of Health, Education and Welfare, Social Security, Administration Children's Bureau.

George Monbiot. 2000. 'Organic Farming Will Feed the World', in *The Guardian*, UK, 24 August.

Ghate, P. 1984. *Direct Attacks on Rural Poverty*. Concept Publications, New Delhi.

Gillin, J.L., Dittmen, C.G., Colbert, R.J. and Kastler, N.M. 1965. *Social Problems*. The Times of India Press, Mumbai.

Goel, Arvind Kumar. 2003. *Orientation in Health Education*. A.B.D. Publishers, Jaipur.

Gore, M.S. 1968. *Urbanization and Family Change*. Popular Prakashan, Bombay.

Green, Reginald Herbold. 1977. *Adult Education in National Development: Planning Notes towards an Integrated Approach*. German Adult Education Association, Bonn.

Gulati, R. and Gulati, K. 2001. *Strengthening Voluntary Action in India: Health and Family Planning Environment*. Konark Publications, New Delhi.

Guru, Mahesh and Chandra, B.P. 1997. 'An Evaluation of Grassroots Level Development Communication System in Karnataka State'. Ph.D. dissertation, Mangalore University.

Guruswamy, M., and Abraham, R.J. 2006. 'Redefining Poverty: A New Poverty Line for a New India', in *Economic Political Weekly*, 24 June, p. 2534–41.

Hermon, Abbon P. 1999. *An Approach to Social Problems.* Ginn Press, Boston.

Hiramani, A.B. 1996. *Health Education*. B.R. Publishing Corp., Delhi.

Jellinek, E.M. 1996. 'Phases in Drinking History of Alcoholics', in *Quarterly Journal of Studies on Alcohol*, June.

Jethithor, Bharat. 2002. *Adult Education and Extension*. A.P.H. Publishing Corp., New Delhi.

Johnson, Elmer H. 1973. *Social Problems of Urban Man.* The Dorsey Press, Homewood, Illinois.

Namjoshi, G.K. 1995. *Health and Population Education*. Nandadeep Prakashan, Ahmedabad.

Kamalth, M.A. 2002. *Home Doctors for India*. D.B. Taraporevala Sons Co. Ltd., Agra.

Kaul, V., Ramchandran, Chitra and Upadhyay, G.C. 1993. *Impact of ECE on Retention in Primary Grades*. National Council of Educational Research and Training, New Delhi.

Keller, Mark and Efron, Vera. 1955. 'The Prevalence of Alcoholism', in *Quarterly Journal of Studies on Alcohol*, December.

Keynes, John Maynard. 2000. 'An Economic Analysis of Unemployment', in *Unemployment as a World Problem*, University of Chicago Press, Chicago.

Khan, A.M. and Bhattacharya, V. 2005. 'Glimpses of Public-Private Old Age Homes: A Pilot Study in Delhi', in *Research and Development Journal*, 11(3), pp. 22–30.

Khanna, R.S. 1996. 'Liberalization and Unemployment in India', in *Journal of Public Administration*, Vol. SLII, July-September.

Kjartan, Renee. 2000. 'Castro Topples Pesticide in Cuba', in *Washington Free Press*, 7 August.

Kothari, Rajani. 1984. 'Communication for Alternative Development: Towards a Paradigm', in *Development Dialogue*, No. 1–2.

Kriesberg, Louis. 1993. 'The Relationship between Socio-Economic Rank and Behaviour', in *Social Problems,* Vol. 10.

Kumar, Anil. 2005. *Health Education*. International Scientific Publishing, New Delhi.

Kumar, B. 1988. *Planning, Development and Poverty Alleviation*. Deep & Deep Publications Pvt. Ltd., New Delhi.

Lakshmi, N.M. 2005. *Health Education and Energy*. Discovery Publication, New Delhi.

Landis, Paul H. 1959. *Social Problems*. J.B. Lippincort Co., Chicago.

Laskin, Richard. 1964. *Social Problems.* McGraw Hill Co., New York.

Lawrence, W.G. and Anderson, C.L. 1986. *Community Health, Times Mirror*. Mosby College Publishing, Missouri.

Lindesmith, Alfred R. 1998. *Opium Addiction.* Principal Press, Bloomington, Indiana.

Lwanga, K.S. and Lemeshow, S. 1991. *Sample Size Determination in Health Studies: A Practical Manual.* World Health Organization, Geneva.

Mahadevan, K. 1992. *Health Education for Quality of Life*. D.K. Publishers, New Delhi.

Mahajan, V.P. 2002. 'Managing Soil Activity for Sustained Production', in *The Tribune* online edition, Chandigarh, 11 March.

Mallick, A. 2006. 'Crime and the Older People', in *Social Welfare*, 8(3), pp. 8–15.

Manja, J.S. 1984. *Health Education and Hygiene*. Universal Publishing, Agra.

Marks, Graham G. et al. 2005. 'Social Projection and Social Conformity in Adolescents Age: A Longitudinal Analysis', in *Personality and Social Psychology Bulletin*, 18(1), pp. 96–101, 19.

Marshall, A. 1957. *Sociology of Deviant Behaviour.* Holt, Rinehart & Winston, New York.

Maslow, R. 1997. 'Social Conformity of Adolescents', in *Perspectives in Psychological Researches*, Vol. 1.7.

McGuire, W.J. 1999. 'Attitude and Attitude Change Regarding Modernization', in *The Handbook of Social Psychology*, 3rd edition, Vol. 2, New York.

McMillen, Wayne. 1995. *Community Organisation for Social Welfare.* University of Chicago Press, Chicago.

McQuail, Denis. 2005. *Mass Communication Theory.* Vistaar Publications, New Delhi.

McVeigh, Frank and Shostak, Arthur. 1978. *Modern Social Problems.* Holt, Rinehart & Winston, New York.

Meredith, Davice. 1990. *Community Health and Social Services.* FFC MDTM, London.

Merton, R.K. and Nisbet, Robert A. (eds). 1971. *Contemporary Social Problems,* Harcourt Brace, New York.

Merton, R.K. 1957. *Social Theory and Social Structure,* Free Press, Glencoe, New York.

Milgram, Lee Kohn. 2005. 'Determinant of Social Conformity: Nationality and Conformity', in *Scientific American*, Vol. 205.

Miller, S.M. and Roby, Pamela. 1970. *The Future of Inequality.* Basic Books, New York.

Ministry of Education and Social Welfare, Directorate of Adult Education. 1973. *Adult Education in India: A Challenge and an Opportunity.* New Delhi.

—— 1974. *National Development: Concepts and Practices in India.* New Delhi.

—— 1979. *Why Should We Become Literate?* New Delhi.

—— 1985. 'Motivational Aspects of the Adult Education Programme', Report of the Motivation Committee. New Delhi.

—— 1987. *Crusade Against Illiteracy: A Collection of Success Stories on Adult Education.* New Delhi.

—— 1987. *Learning for Participation: An Approach to Training in Adult Education.* New Delhi.

—— 1988. *Literacy and Learning: Some Thoughts on Education*. New Delhi.

Ministry of Social Justice and Empowerment. 'National Policy for Older Persons', from http: //socialjustice.nic.in/social/sdcop/npop.pdf.

Ministry of Water Resources. 2002. 'National Water Policy'. Government of India, p. 18.

Mishra, R.C. 2005. *Health Nutrition Education*. A.P.H. Publishing Corp., New Delhi.

Misra, B.D. 1980. *Introduction to the Study of Population*. South Asia Publishers, New Delhi.

Mittal, M. 1992. *Child Labour in Unorganized Sector*. Sterling Publishers, New Delhi.

Mohan, D. 1980. *Drug Abuse in India*, AIIMS, Delhi.

Mohanty, Jagannath. 2000. *Adult and Non-Formal Education*. Deep & Deep Publications Pvt. Ltd., New Delhi.

Mundt, C. 2000. 'Genetic Diversity and Disease Control in Rice', in *Nature*, 406, pp. 718–22.

Mutthirulandi, Raja. 'Globalization and Education, Need for Curriculum for Lifelong Learning Programmes'. *www.boloji.com*.

Myrdal, Gunnar. 1990. *Population*. Harvard University Press, Cambridge, Massachusetts.

Nanda, V.K. 2000. *Health Education*. Anmol Publications, New Delhi.

National Workshop on Implementation of Environmental Legislations for Protection and Conservation of Environment. 2003. 12–16 October.

Neumeyer, M.H. 1953. *Social Problems and the Changing Society*. Princeton, New Jersey.

Nortman, Dorothy L. 1975. 'A Longitudinal Analysis of Population Policies in Developing Countries', in R.K. Godwin (ed.): *Comparative Policy Analysis*, D.C. Heath, Lexington.

NSSO. 2002. '58th Round of NSSO Survey on Disabled Persons in India'. Ministry of Statistics and Programme Implementation, New Delhi.

Ornati, Oscar. 1964. 'Poverty in America', quoted by Howard Becker in *Social Problems*.

Pandey, G.P. 1999. *Press and Social Change*. Manak Publications, New Delhi.

Patel, M. and Kamala, R. 1994. 'Situation of Institutionalized and Non-Institutionalized Aging Women', in *Indian Journal of Gerontology*, 9(182), pp. 25–50.

Paul, B. and Leslie, Gerald R. 1970. *The Sociology and Social Problem*. Appleton Century Crofts, New York, 4th edition.

Pejaver, R.K. and Nair, M.K.C. 2001. *Adolescent Care 2000 and Beyond*. Prism Books Pvt. Ltd., Bangalore.

Peter, Rosset M. 1999. 'The Multiple Functions and Benefits of Small Farm Agriculture in the Context of Global Trade Negotiations'. Policy brief prepared for 'Cultivating Our Futures', the FAO/Netherlands Conference on the Multifunctional Character of Agriculture and Land, Maastricht, The Netherlands, 12–17 September.

Prakash, I. 1999. *Ageing in India*. World Health Organization, Geneva.

Raab, Earl and Selznick, G.J. 1959. *Major Social Problems*. Row Peterson & Co. Illinois.

Rai, B.C. 2002. *Health Education and Hygiene*. Prakashan Kendra, New Delhi.

Rajani, R. Shirur. 1990. *Reproductive and Sexual Health Education for Adolescents Needs Assessment*. Discovery Publications House, New Delhi.

Ram, Chandran L. and Dharmaliy T. 1986. *Health Education: A New Approach*. Vikas Publication, New Delhi.

Rao, P.S. and Inderaj, S.C. 1970. *Journal of Family Welfare*, Vol. XVII, Family Planning Association of India, Mumbai, June.

Rao, Rama Mohan, Batchelor, C.H., James, A.J., Nagaraja, R., Seeley, J. and Butterworth, J.A. (eds). 2003. 'Andhra Pradesh Rural Livelihoods Programme: Water Resources Audit Phase 1 Report'. APRLP, Hyderabad.

Reddy, M.M.K. 2000. *Health and Family Welfare*. Kanishka Publishers & Distributors, New Delhi.

Rehabilitation Council of India. 2004. 'Report on Manpower Development'. Delhi.

Reinhardt, James M., Meadows, Paul and Gillette, John M. 1952. *Social Problems and Social Policy*. American Book Co., New York.

Rose, Arnold. 1957. 'Theory for the Study of Social Problems', in *Social Problems*.

Ross, Aileen. 1961. *Hindu Family in its Urban Setting*. Oxford University Press, New Delhi.

Ross, Peter H. and Blum, Zahava D. 1967. *Class, Status and Poverty*. Basic Books, New York.

Roy, Nikhil Ranjan. 2004. *Adult Education in India and Abroad*. S. Chandar & Corp., New Delhi.

Sabatini, A.C. 2002. 'Whom Do International Donors Support in the Name of Civil Society?', in *Development in Practice*, 12(1), pp. 7–19.

Sagar, Deep. 1990. 'Rural Development Policies of India: A Historical Analysis', in *The Indian Journal of Public Administration,* Delhi, Vol. 36, No. 2.

Sen, Amit. 2005. *Health Education and Nutrition*. Isha Books, New Delhi.

Sharma, Inder Prabha. 2001. *Adult Education in India*. N.B.O. Publishers Distributors, New Delhi.

Sharma, K. 1999. *Tea Industry in India: An Introduction*. N.L. Publishers, Dibrugarh, Assam, p. 16.

Shepard, J.M. and Voss, H.L. 1978. *Social Problems*. Macmillan Publishing Co. Inc., New York.

Sherry, G.P. 1963. *Health Education*. Popular Press, Agra.

Shrivastava, S.L. 1987. *Five Year Plans and Economic Growth*. Deep & Deep Publications Pvt. Ltd., New Delhi.

Sidhu, R.S. and Dhillon, M.S. 1997. 'Land and Water Resources in Punjab: Their Degradation and Technologies for Sustainable Use', in *Indian Journal of Agricultural Economics*, Vol. 52, No. 3, p. 510.

Singh, U.K. and Nayak, A.K. 1997. *Health Education*. Commonwealth Publishers, New Delhi.

Singh, Yogendra. 2000. *Cultural Change in India: Identity and Globalization*. Rawat Publications, Jaipur, New Delhi.

Sinha, R.K. 1988. *Economic Development since Independence*. Deep & Deep Publications Pvt. Ltd., New Delhi.

Smith, C.E. 1994. *Health Instruction Year Book*. Stanford University, Oxford.

Social Work Year Books, Vols. 1–9 (1929–97). Russel Sage Foundation, New York.

Stark, Rodney. 1975. *Social Problems.* Random House, New York.

Stephenson, L.S., Latham, M.C. and Ottesen, E.A. 2000. 'Malnutrition and Parasitic Helminthes Infections', in *Parasitology*, 121 (suppl.) pp. S23–8.

Subrahmanya, R.K.A. 2002. 'Social Security for the Elderly', in *Research and Development Journal*, 5(3), pp. 22–30.

Tabish, A. 2000. *The Future of Health*. Paras Publishing Pvt. Ltd., New Delhi.

Tandon, R. 2001. 'Citizenship, Participation and Accountability: A Perspective', in *Innovations in Civil Society*, 1(1), pp. 17–22.

The World Bank Working Paper Series. 1989. World Bank, Washington.

Tripathy, S.N. 1997. *Migrant Child Labour in India*. Mohit Publications, New Delhi.

United Nations Economic and Social Commission for Asia and the Pacific (www.unescap.org).

Uphoff, N. 1995. 'Grass Roots Organizations & NGOs in Rural Development: Opportunities with Diminishing States and Expanding Markets', in A. De Janvry, E. Sadoqulet, S. Radwan, and E. Thorbecke (eds): *State, Market and Civil Organizations.* Macmillan Press, London, pp. 168–97.

Vardappan, S. 2002. *Population Information, Education and Communication*. A.V.P. Publisher, New Delhi.

Veeresh, G.K. 1998. 'Organic Farming: Ecologically Sound and Economically Sustainable', in *Man and Development*, March.

Verghese, B.G. 2001. 'Education, Media and Society', in *Mainstream*, 22 December.

Waskin, Richard (ed.). 1964. *Social Problems.* McGraw Hill & Co., New York.

Weber, Max. 1961. 'The Urban Community', in *Theories of Society*, Vol. 1, The Free Press of Glencoe, New York.

Wilson, Charles. 1987. *Health Education: A Guide for Teachers and a Textbook*. Teachers Education, Washington.

World Health Organization. 1992. 'Comprehensive School Health Education: Suggested Guidelines for Action', in WHO/UNESCO/Unicef unpublished document. Division of Health Education and Promotion, WHO, Geneva.

World Health Organization. 2002. 'Health and Ageing: A Discussion Paper'. WHO, Geneva.

World Health Organization. 2002. 'World Health Report 2002: Reducing Risks, Promoting Healthy Life'. WHO, Geneva.

Yadava, J.S. 1995. *Media for the Masses*. Department of Journalism and Mass Communication, Banaras Hindu University, Varanasi.

Zhang, J.I.E. 2000. 'Modernizations, Interpersonal Power and Conformity: A Cross-Cultural Study of Significant Others' Influence on Adolescents', Ph.D. thesis, Brigham Young University, Hawai, USA.

Webliography

Webliography (All these website was accessed between 2005–2008)

'Globalization and the Incorporation of Education'. Available at www.infed.org.

'Globalization of Education in the Americas'. Available at http://www.vcn.bc.ca/idea/kuehn./htm.

http://mohfw.nic.in/dofw%20website/Child%20healthrti.pdf

http://www.aahperd.org/iejhe/2005/sharma.pdf

http://www.newdelhi.usebassy.goy/hiypolicy/html

http://www.pubmedcentral.nih.gov/pagerender.fcgi?artid-1527844&pageindex=1

http://www.searo.who.int/en/Section313/Section1519_10855xc.html

http://www.vhai.org/htm/hp/health_promotion.asp

http://member.aahperd.org/iejhe/template.cfm?template=2005/sharma.html.

http://planning.kar.nic.in/AP0506Volume%20I/AP0506-Colum%20I/chapter17.doc

org.in/rights/pressmanual/rightsofaged.htm

Ramaya, K. 'Rights of the Aged'. Available at http://www.britishcouncil.

www.mohfw.nic.in/NRHM%20state%20and%20district%20health % 20mission-instit

www.mohfw.nic.in/NRHM%state%20anddistrict%20health%20mission-institutional%20setup.htm-489k

Index